HESI Live Review Workbook for the NCLEX-RN Exam

Rosemary Pine, PhD, RN, BC, CDE
Director, Review Courses
Elsevier Review and Testing
Nursing and Health Professions
Houston, Texas

Sandra L. Upchurch, PhD, RN
Former Director Curriculum
Elsevier Review and Testing
Nursing and Health Professions
Houston, Texas

Traci Henry, MSN, RN
Curriculum Manager
Elsevier Review and Testing
Nursing and Health Professions
Houston, Texas

Marilyn Tompkins, DrPH, RN, FNP, BC
Family Nurse Practitioner
Lakeside-Milam Recovery Centers
Kirkland, Washington

Jo-Anne Gaudet, MSN, RN, CCRN
Clinical Educator
Houston Methodist Hospital
Houston, Texas

Judy Siefert, MSN, RN
Director, Testing
Elsevier Review and Testing
Nursing and Health Professions
Houston, Texas

The editors and publisher would also like to acknowledge the following individuals for contributions to the previous editions of this book.

Susan Morrison, PhD, RN, FAAN
President Emerita
Elsevier Review and Testing
Nursing and Health Professions
Houston, Texas

Ainslie Nibert, PhD, RN, FAAN
Former Senior
Vice President
Elsevier Review and Testing
Nursing and Health Professions
Houston, Texas

Mickie Hinds, PhD, RN
Former Director, Review and Curriculum
Elsevier Review and Testing
Nursing and Health Professions
Houston, Texas

Judy Siefert, MSN, RN
Director, Testing
Elsevier Review and Testing
Houston, Texas

Denise Voyles, MS, RN
Testing Manager
Elsevier Review and Testing
Nursing and Health Professions
Houston, Texas

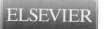

ELSEVIER

3251 Riverport Lane
St. Louis, MO 63043

ISBN: 978-0-323-39635-6

2014-2015 HESI Live
Review Workbook for the NCLEX-RN Exam, Revised Reprint

NOTICE

Knowledge and best practice in the field of nursing are constantly changing. As new research and experience broaden our understanding, changes in research methods, professional practices, or medical treatment may become necessary.

Practitioners and researchers must always rely on their own experience and knowledge in evaluating and using any information, methods, compounds, or experiments described herein. In using such information or methods, they should be mindful of their own safety and the safety of others, including parties for whom they have a professional responsibility.

With respect to any drug or pharmaceutical products identified, readers are advised to check the most current information provided (i) on procedures featured or (ii) by the manufacturer of each product to be administered, to verify the recommended dose or formula, the method and duration of administration, and contraindications. It is the responsibility of practitioners, relying on their own experience and knowledge of their clients, to make diagnoses, to determine dosages and the best treatment for each individual client, and to take all appropriate safety precautions.

To the fullest extent of the law, neither the Publisher nor the authors, contributors, or editors assume any liability for any injury and/or damage to persons or property as a matter of products liability, negligence, or otherwise, or from any use or operation of any methods, products, instructions, or ideas contained in the material herein.

The Publisher

NCLEX®, NCLEX-RN®, and NCLEX-PN® are registered trademarks of the National Council of State Boards of Nursing, Inc.

NANDA International Nursing Diagnoses: Definitions and Classifications 2012-2014; Herdman T.H. (ED); copyright © 2012, 1994-2012 NANDA International; published by John Wiley & Sons, Limited.

International Standard Book Number: 978-0-323-39635-6

Executive Content Strategist: Kristin Geen
Associate Content Development Specialist: Laura Goodrich
Publishing Services Manager: Jeff Patterson
Senior Project Manager: Anne Konopka
Designer: Karen Pauls

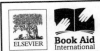

Working together
to grow libraries in
developing countries

www.elsevier.com • www.bookaid.org

Printed in the United States of America

Last digit is the print number: 9 8 7 6 5 4 3 2

Test-Taking Strategies and Study Guide

Welcome To The Hesi Live Review Course

This series of slides and the workbook provide test-taking strategies, sample test questions, and a content review of the nursing curriculum to help prepare nursing students for the NCLEX-RN examination. For a more in-depth review of certain material, please refer to the following:

- *HESI Comprehensive Review for the NCLEX-RN Examination*
- *Mosby's Comprehensive Review of Nursing for the NCLEX-RN Examination*
- *HESI/Saunders Online Review for the NCLEX-RN Examination*

Knowledge is power!

Goals of the Live Review Course

- Strengthen test-taking skills
- Incorporate recommended strategies to manage anxiety
- Formulate a study plan using tools such as the HESI Live Review Workbook for the NCLEX-RN Exam
- Review basic curriculum content

NLCEX-RN Examination

About the NCLEX-RN Blueprint

- The tests cover essential nursing knowledge.
- The test plan is revised every 3 years after a practice analysis has been conducted with entry-level nurses.
- Information about the test plan, including descriptions of content categories and related content for each category, can be found on the website for the National Council of State Boards of Nursing *(www.ncsbn.org)*.
- The NCSBN website also presents information for students, frequently asked questions, and examples of alternate formats.
- The content of the NCLEX-RN Test Plan is organized into four major client needs categories. Two of the four categories are divided into subcategories:
  — Safe and Effective Care Environment
    • Management of Care
    • Safety and Infection Control
  — Health Promotion and Maintenance
  — Psychosocial Integrity
  — Physiological Integrity
    • Basic Care and Comfort
    • Pharmacological and Parenteral Therapies
    • Reduction of Risk Potential
    • Physiological Adaptation

[handwritten note:] Studying for NCLEX: 1500 - 3000 questions 30 hrs. per week

Processes

Processes fundamental to RN practice are integrated into all client needs categories.

- Nursing process
  - Planning and implementing nursing care based on assessment, diagnosis, and determining priorities
  - Evaluating the effectiveness of nursing care
- Caring
- Communication and documentation
- Teaching and learning

About Test Administration

With computerized adaptive testing (CAT), the difficulty of the exam is tailored to the candidate's ability level.

All RN candidates must answer a minimum of 75 items. The maximum number of items the candidate may answer during the allotted 6-hour period is ~~265~~. 265. ~~265~~

[handwritten margin note: Avg. # of questions: 118. 15 of first 75 are experimental]

About Test Item Questions

Multiple choice items

- Comprise the majority of items
- One question with four choices (answers) from which to choose the correct response

Multiple response items

- Require the candidate to select one or more than one response from five to seven choices
- The candidate is instructed to select all that apply

[handwritten margin note: At least 2, but never all are correct.]

Fill-in-the-blank items

- Require a candidate to type in one or more numbers in a calculation item
- If rounding is necessary, it is performed at the end of the calculation

Hot spot items

- Instruct the candidate to identify one or more areas on a picture or graphic
- Can measure skills related to safety, physical assessment, and other procedures and techniques

Chart/exhibit format

- Presents the candidate with a problem that requires the individual to read the information in the chart/exhibit to arrive at the answer
- Provides the client history, laboratory data, and clinical data on tabs

Ordered response items or drag and drop

- Require a candidate to rank order or move options to provide the correct answer
- Presents the candidate with a list of the essential steps of a nursing procedure (e.g., CPR) and instructs the individual to order the steps in the correct sequence

Audio item format
- Presents the candidate with an audio clip; the individual uses headphones to listen to the question and select the answer option that applies
- Evaluates the candidate's competence in certain skills or assessment areas

Graphic options
- May be used as all or part of an individual item, either in the question itself or as part of the response

Test-Taking Strategies

General Strategies
- Every question must be answered to move to the next question, so make your best guess if you are not sure of the answer.
- Quickly eliminate the options that do not answer the question.
- Reread the question for qualifiers or other words that specify what the question asks.
- Decide what makes the responses different from each other.
- Keep in mind that the choice may contain correct information but may not answer the question.

For Your Toolbox
- Use the *ABC*s when selecting an answer or determining the order of priority.
  - Remember the order of priority: airway, breathing, and circulation.
  - The exception to the rule, which is with actual CPR, is C-A-B.
- *Maslow's Hierarchy of Needs*
  - Address physiological needs first, followed by safety and security needs, love and belonging needs, self-esteem needs and, finally, self-actualization needs.
  - When a physiological need is not addressed in the question, look for the option that addresses safety.
- Carefully read the question to determine the step of the nursing process.
  - *Assessment* questions address the gathering and verification of data.
  - *Analysis* questions require the nurse to:
    - Interpret data and collect additional information
    - Identify and communicate nursing diagnoses
    - Determine the health team's ability to meet the client's needs
  - *Planning* questions ask about determining, prioritizing, and modifying outcomes of care.
  - *Implementation* questions reflect the management and organization of care and the assignment and delegation of tasks. Be prepared for questions on client teaching.
  - *Evaluation* questions focus on comparing the actual outcomes of care with the expected outcomes and on communicating and documenting findings.

(handwritten notes)
- Start w/ least invasive intervention
- Assess before taking action, when appropriate
- Have necessary information/take all relevant actions before calling provider
- Which client to assess first
- Client before equipment
- Follow guidelines for delegation

- Think: safety, safety, SAFETY!
- Start with the least invasive intervention.
- Assess before taking action, when appropriate.
- Have all necessary information and take all possible relevant actions before calling the physician/healthcare provider.
- Determine which client to assess first (i.e., most at risk, most physiologically unstable).
- Follow guidelines for delegating assignments. Remember the differences between the role of the licensed nurse and the role of unlicensed assistive personnel (UAP).

The Question May Contain "Red Flag" Words

Practice rewording the following questions:
1. "Which response indicates to the nurse a need to reteach the client about …"
2. "Which prescription (order) should the nurse question?"

Common Interventions
- Small, frequent feedings
- Recommended fluid intake: "3 L/day"
- Alternate rest with activity
- Conserve energy with any activity

Teaching Points
- Risk factors—known modifiable versus nonmodifiable
- Prevention and wellness promotion
- New medications/self-care instructions
- Client empowerment
- Anticipatory guidance
- Incorporating client education information into the client's lifestyle, culture, spiritual beliefs, and so on

A Few Words About "Words"

Healthcare provider (HCP): The person prescribing care (e.g., physician, nurse practitioner)

Prescriptions: Orders written by licensed healthcare providers

Unlicensed assistive personnel (UAP)
- Client care technician
- Nursing assistant
- Nurse's aide

Keep Memorizing to a Minimum
- Growth and developmental milestones
- Death and dying stages
- Crisis intervention
- Immunizations
- Drug classifications
- Principles of teaching/learning
- Stages of pregnancy and fetal growth
- Nurse Practice Act: Standards of Practice and Delegation

Practice Rewording

1. _____

2. _____

Strategies for Success in Answering NCLEX-RN Questions: Four Essential Steps

1. Determine whether the style of the question is

    + positive +

    or

    − negative −

2. Find the key words in the question.
3. Rephrase the question in your own words and then answer the question.
4. Rule out options.

Determine Whether the Question Is Written in a Positive or Negative Style

- A *positive style* may ask what the nurse should do, or the best or first action to implement.
- A *negative style* may ask what the nurse should avoid, which prescription the nurse should question, or which behavior indicates the need for reteaching the client.

Find the Key Words in the Question

- Ask yourself which words or phrases provide the critical information.
- This information may be the age of the client, the setting, the timing, a set of symptoms or behaviors, or any number of other factors.
- For example, the nursing actions for a 10-year-old, 1-day postoperative client are different from those for a 70-year-old, 1-hour postoperative client.

Rephrase the Question in Your Own Words and Answer the Question

- This will help you to eliminate nonessential information in the question and to determine the correct answer.
- Ask yourself, "What is this instructor *really* asking?"
- Before looking at the choices, rephrase the question in your own words.
- Answer the question.

Rule Out Options

- Based on your knowledge, you can probably identify one or two options that are clearly incorrect.
- Mentally mark through those options on the computer monitor.
- Now, differentiate between the remaining options, considering your knowledge of the subject and related nursing principles, such as the roles of the nurse, the nursing process, the ABCs, and Maslow's Hierarchy of Needs.

A hospitalized client reports to the nurse that he has not had a bowel movement in 2 days. Which intervention should the nurse implement first?

A. Instruct the caregiver to offer a glass of warm prune juice at mealtimes.
B. Notify the healthcare provider and request a prescription for a stool softener.
C. Assess the client's medical record to determine his normal bowel pattern. *(least invasive)*
D. Instruct the caregiver to increase the client's fluids to five 8-ounce glasses per day.

[handwritten: C circled]

HESI Test Question Approach

Positive?		**YES** *(circled)*	NO
Key Words	*first/priority*		

Rephrase

Rule Out Choices

~~A~~	B	C	~~D~~

These are similar.

A client who has COPD is resting in a semi-Fowler's position with oxygen at 2 L/min per nasal cannula. The client develops dyspnea. What action should the RN take first?

A. Call the healthcare provider.
B. Obtain a bedside pulse oximeter.
C. Raise the head of the bed higher.
D. Assess the client's vital signs.

[handwritten: C circled]

HESI Test Question Approach

Positive?		**YES** *(circled)*	NO
Key Words	*dyspnea* *position (45 degrees)*		

Rephrase

Rule Out Choices

A	~~B~~	C	~~D~~

does not help client breathe better; similar

Specific Areas of Content

Laboratory Values

Know the normal ranges for commonly used laboratory tests, what variations mean, and the *best* nursing actions.

- H & H
- WBC, RBC, platelets
- Electrolytes: K^+, Na^+, Ca^{2+}, Mg^{2+}, Cl^-, PO_4
- BUN and creatinine
- Relationship of Ca^{2+} and PO_4
- ABGs
- PT, INR, PTT (don't get them confused)

A client who has hyperparathyroidism is scheduled to receive a prescribed dose of oral phosphate. The RN notes that the client's serum calcium level is 12.5 mg/dL. What action should the nurse take? *[handwritten: ↑ H]*

A. Hold the phosphate and notify the healthcare provider.
B. Review the client's serum parathyroid hormone level.
C. Give a PRN dose of IV calcium per protocol.
D. Administer the dose of oral phosphate.

[handwritten: D circled]

phosphate low when calcium is high

HESI Test Question Approach

Positive?		**YES** *(circled)*	NO
Key Words	*calcium level* *action*		

Rephrase

Rule Out Choices

A	~~B~~	~~C~~	D

not necessary   *Ca⁺ already high.*

In completing a client's preoperative routine, the RN finds that the operative permit has not been signed. The client begins to ask more questions about the surgical procedure. What action should the nurse take next?

A. Witness the client's signature on the permit.
B. Answer the client's questions about the surgery.
C. Inform the healthcare provider that the client has questions about the surgery.
D. Reassure the client that the surgeon will answer any questions before the anesthetic is administered.

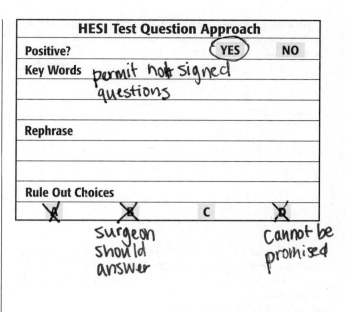

HESI Test Question Approach				
Positive?			YES	NO
Key Words	permit not signed questions			
Rephrase				
Rule Out Choices				
	⨉A	⨉B	C	⨉D

surgeon should answer

cannot be promised

Nutrition

- Be able to identify foods relative to their sodium content (high or low), potassium level (high or low), and increased levels of phosphate, iron, or vitamin K
- Chemotherapy, GI/GU disturbances
- Proteins, CHOs, fats
- Pregnancy and fetal growth needs
- Remember these concepts:
  — Introducing one food at a time (infants, allergies) → single source foods
  — Progression "AS TOLERATED" (N/V?) → check appetite
  - The nursing assessment that guides decisions about progression

Medication Administration and Pharmacology

Pharmacological treatment and related nursing implications are reviewed in each chapter to coincide with the disease processes and conditions of the client.

More critical thinking questions are being designed around SKILLS!

Think: safety, *safety,* SAFETY!

Reflect on … the *whole picture.*

Safe medication administration is more than just knowing the action of the medications. It also includes:
- The "6 Rights" (six *plus* technique of skill execution)
  1. Right drug
  2. Right dose
  3. Right route
  4. Right time
  5. Right patient
  6. Right documentation
- Drug interactions
- Vulnerable organs (√ labs; what to assess) → most drugs metabolized in liver
- Allergies and presence of suprainfections
- Concept of peak and trough

How you would know:
- Whether the drug is working
- A problem has arisen

Teaching: *safety, empowerment, compliance*

Special Considerations

- Teratogens
- Vesicants
- Implications of edema, impaired tissue perfusion at injection site
- Relationship of hepatorenal status to drug dose/frequency
- Concepts of weaning

Practical Tips

When answering an NCLEX question:

Do not respond based on …

- *Your* past client care experiences or agency
- A familiar phrase or term
- "Of course, *I* would have already …"
- What *you* think is *realistic*
- *Your* children, pregnancies, parents, elders, personal response to a drug, and so on

Do respond based on …

- ABCs
- Scientific, behavioral, sociological principles
- Principles of teaching/learning
- Maslow's Hierarchy of Needs
- Nursing process
- Answer based only on what the questions asks no more, no less
- NCLEX-RN ideal hospital
- Basic A & P
- Critical thinking

Best Practice for a Successful NCLEX-RN Exam

Manage Anxiety Between Now and the Test

- Think positively and believe in yourself.
- Use positive self-talk ("I can do this!")
- Do set up a study schedule and stick to it.
- Do avoid negative people.
- Do respect your body and your mind.
- Do establish a balanced lifestyle (i.e., a regular schedule for sleeping, eating, exercising, socializing, and working).

Develop a Study Schedule

- Organize resources.
  - Online texts, hard copy books, review questions
  - Practice tests, case studies
- Identify your challenges; review these:
  - Results of your HESI Exit Exam
  - Final grades
  - Feedback on clinical performance
  - Results of practice tests
- Initially take practice tests specific to your areas of weakness.
- Establish a study schedule that includes adequate time to prepare.

- Know your testing date.
  — Plan your schedule for the 4 to 8 weeks before your testing date.
- Would a study group help you?
- Make sure you have a comfortable level of memorization of growth and development markers, lab results, drug categories, drug calculations, and immunization schedules.

A Week before the Exam
- Take a test drive to the site.
- Be mindful of traffic patterns.
- Familiarize yourself with the test center.
- Confirm that you have all the documents you need to be admitted to the exam.

The Day Before the Test
- Do allow only 30 minutes to review test-taking strategies.
- If you feel the need to, review your notes the night before the exam, but allow for a restful 7 to 8 hours of sleep.
- Do assemble all necessary materials:
  — Admission ticket
  — Directions to testing center
  — Identification
  — Money for lunch
- Do something you enjoy.
- Do respect your body and your mind.

The Day of the Test
- Eat a healthy meal.
- Do allow plenty of time to get to the testing center.
- Do dress comfortably.
- Do take only your identification forms into the testing room.
- Do avoid distractions.
- Do use positive self-talk.

At the Exam
- Breathe deeply and regularly.
- Continue the positive self-talk.
- Be in the moment and take the exam; no regrets.
- Do not allow the number of questions to influence your level of self-confidence.

You can do this!

2 Legal Aspects and Clinical Management of Care

Legal Aspects

Legal Systems
- Civil law is concerned with the protection of the client's private rights.
- Criminal law deals with the rights of individuals and society as defined by legislative laws.

Nursing negligence is the failure to exercise the proper degree of care required by the circumstances that a reasonably prudent person would exercise under the circumstances to avoid harming others. It is a careless act of omission or commission that results in injury to another.

Nursing malpractice, often referred to as *professional negligence,* is a type of negligence. It is the failure to use that degree of care that a reasonable nurse would use under the same or similar circumstances.

Malpractice is found when:
- The nurse owed a duty to the client.
- The nurse did not carry out that duty or breached that duty.
- The client was injured.
- The nurse's failure to carry out that duty caused the client's injury.

Standards of Care
- Nurses are required to follow standards of care, which originate in Nurse Practice Acts, state and federal law (US) and provincial, territorial, and federal laws (Canada), accreditation recommendations, the guidelines of professional organizations, and the written policies and procedures of the healthcare agency.
- Nurses are responsible for performing procedures correctly and exercising professional judgment when implementing healthcare providers' prescriptions.

The unlicensed assistive personnel (UAP) reports to a staff nurse that a client, who had surgery 4 hours ago has had a decrease in blood pressure (BP), from 150/80 to 110/70, in the past hour. The nurse advises the UAP to check the client's dressing for excess drainage and report the findings to the nurse. Which factor is most important to consider when assessing the legal ramifications of this situation?
- A. The parameters of the state's or province's nurse practice act.
- B. The need to complete an adverse occurrence report.
- C. Hospital protocols regarding the frequency of vital sign assessment every hour postoperatively.
- D. The health care provider's prescription for changing the postoperative dressing.

inappropriate delegation

HESI Test Question Approach			
Positive?		YES	NO
Key Words	UAP		
	Dressing		
Rephrase			
Rule Out Choices			
A	B	C	D

In the elevator the UAP overhears two nurses talking about a client who will lose her leg because of the negligence of the staff. What federal law has been violated?

(A) Health Insurance Portability and Accountability Act (HIPAA)
B. Americans with Disabilities Act (ADA)
C. Nurse Practice Act (NPA)
D. Patient Self-Determination Act (PSDA)

HESI Test Question Approach			
Positive?		YES	NO
Key Words	Overhears violated		
Rephrase			
Rule Out Choices			
A	~~B~~	C	~~D~~

Practice Issues

■ Nurses must follow the healthcare provider's prescription unless the nurse believes that it is in error; that it violates hospital policy; or that it is harmful to the client.
■ The nurse makes a formal report explaining the refusal.
■ The nurse should file an incident (occurrence) report for any situation that may result in harm to the client.

Advance Directives (ADs)

■ Assess the client's knowledge of advance directives.
■ Integrate them into the client's plan of care.
■ Provide the client with information about advance directives or review ADs on admission.
■ Advance directives can limit life-prolonging measures when there is little or no chance of recovery.
■ Living will—A client documents his or her wishes regarding future care in the event of terminal illness.
■ Durable power of attorney for healthcare—A client appoints a representative (healthcare proxy) to make healthcare decisions.
— The client must receive AD information or review ADs on admission.
— Living wills and advance directives (Canada)
• Instructional advance directives—gives directions on the level of health interventions.
• Proxy directive—names a substitute decision maker
• Advance Directives are evolving and vary throughout the provinces and territories

An awake and alert client with impending pulmonary edema is brought to the emergency department. The client provides the nurse with a copy of a living will that states that "no invasive" medical procedures should be used to "keep her alive." The healthcare team is questioning whether the client should be intubated. What information should guide the team's decision?

A. The living will removes the obligation to involve the client in any medical decision making.
(B.) The client is awake and alert, which makes the living will irrelevant and nonbinding.
C. Lifesaving measures do not need to be explained to the client because of the signed living will.
D. The family should be contacted to determine who has durable power of attorney for health care for the client.

HESI Test Question Approach			
Positive?		YES	NO
Key Words			
Rephrase			
Rule Out Choices			
A	B	C	D

living will in place when pt. not alert/awake

Restraints/Safety Reminder Devices (SRDs)

- Restraints and SRDs can be used *only:*
  - To ensure the physical safety of the client or other residents
  - When less restrictive interventions are not successful
  - On the written order of a healthcare provider
- The nurse must follow agency policy and procedure to restrain any client.
- Documentation of the use of restraints and of follow-up assessments must detail the attempts to use less restrictive interventions.
- Liability for improper or unlawful restraint lies with the nurse and the healthcare facility.

[handwritten: LAST RESORT]

[handwritten: hydration, skin integrity, toileting, N/V (risk for aspiration), circulation]

A family member of a client who is in a Posey vest restraint (SRD) asks why the restraint was applied. How should the nurse respond?

A. The restraint was prescribed by the healthcare provider.
B. There are not enough staff members to keep the client safe all the time.
C. The other clients are upset when the client wanders at night.
D. The client's actions place her at high risk for harming herself.

[handwritten: doesn't answer question]
[handwritten: not appropriate]

HESI Test Question Approach			
Positive?		(YES)	NO
Key Words			
Rephrase			
Rule Out Choices			
~~A~~	~~B~~	~~C~~	D

Legal Aspects of Mental Health

- Admissions
  - Involuntary
  - Emergency
- Client's rights
- Competency

What nursing action has the highest priority when admitting a client to a psychiatric unit on an involuntary basis?

A. Reassure the client that the admission is only for a limited time.
B. Offer the client and family the opportunity to share their feelings about the admission.
C. Determine the behaviors that resulted in the need for admission. *[handwritten: ♥ meet physiological needs]*
D. Advise the client about the legal rights of all hospitalized clients.

HESI Test Question Approach			
Positive?		(YES)	NO
Key Words	*highest priority involuntary*		
Rephrase			
Rule Out Choices			
~~A~~	~~B~~	C	D

[handwritten: up Maslow's hierarchy]

Confidential Health Care

- The Health Insurance Portability and Accountability Act of 1996 (HIPAA) established standards for the verbal, written and electronic exchange of private health information.
- HIPAA created clients' rights to consent to use and disclose health information, to inspect and copy one's medical record, and to amend mistaken or incomplete information.
- HIPAA requires all hospitals and health agencies to have specific policies and procedures in place to ensure compliance with its standards.

The **Personal Information Protection and Electronic Documents Act (PIPEDA) (Canada)** is federal legislation that protects personal information, including health information. PIPEDA delineates how private-sector organizations may collect, use, or disclose personal information.

Informed Consent

Informed consent must meet the following criteria:
- The client giving consent is competent and of legal age.
- The consent is given voluntarily.
    — The client giving consent understands the procedure, its risks and benefits, and alternative procedures.
- The client giving consent has the right to have all questions answered satisfactorily.
- It is the duty of the healthcare provider who is performing the procedure or treatment to obtain informed consent.
- The RN is witnessing the signature, not providing informed consent.
- Answers to any questions the client has about a procedure are the responsibility of the healthcare provider who will perform the procedure.

The nurse enters the room of a preoperative client to obtain the client's signature on the surgical consent form. Which question is most important for the nurse to ask the client?
A. "When did the surgeon explain the procedure to you?"
B. "Is any member of your family going to be here during your surgery?"
C. "Have you been instructed in postoperative activities and restrictions?"
D. "Have you received any preoperative pain medication?"

Competency to sign

Good Samaritan Laws

- Good Samaritan laws limit liability if a nurse offers assistance at the scene of an accident, as long as the nurse acts within acceptable standards of care.
- The nurse should provide only care that is consistent with his or her level of expertise.

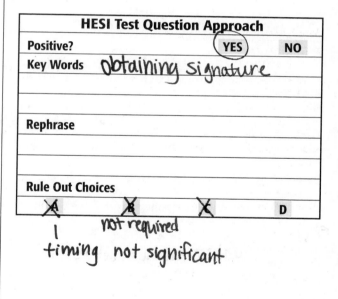

HESI Test Question Approach

HESI Test Question Approach		
Positive?	YES	NO
Key Words	obtaining signature	
Rephrase		
Rule Out Choices		
A B C		D

not required
timing not significant

Practice within scope of nursing practice
Do not move unless risk of fine

Abuse

- The nurse has legal responsibilities related to reporting incidences of abuse, neglect, or violence.
- Healthcare professionals who do not report suspected abuse or neglect are liable for civil or criminal legal action.

Which assignment should the nurse delegate to a UAP in an acute care setting?
A. Hourly blood glucose checks for a client with a continuous insulin drip.
B. Giving PO medications left at the bedside for the client to take after eating.
C. Taking vital signs for an older client with left humeral and left tibial fractures.
D. Replacing a client's pressure ulcer dressing that has been soiled by incontinence.

Clinical Management of Care

Communication Skills

Types of leadership:
- *"Do it my way."*
  — Aggressive communication/authoritarian leader
- *"Whatever ... as long as you like me."*
  — Passive communication/laissez-faire leader
- *"Let's consider the options available."*
  — Assertive communication/democratic leader

The charge nurse confronts a staff nurse whose behavior has been resentful and negative since a change in unit policy was announced. The staff nurse states, "Don't blame me; nobody likes this idea." What is the charge nurse's priority action?
A. Confront the other staff members involved in the change of unit policy.
B. Call a unit meeting to review the reasons the change was made.
C. Develop a written unit policy for the expression of complaints.
D. Encourage the nurse to be accountable for her own behavior. *address conduct before meeting.*

Delegation Skills

Delegation is the process by which responsibility and authority—but *not* accountability— are transferred to another individual.
- The nursing process or any activity requiring nursing judgment may not be delegated to the UAP (UCP).
- Five rights of delegation
  — Right task
  — Right circumstance
  — Right person
  — Right direction/communication
  — Right supervision

HESI Test Question Approach

Positive?		YES	NO
Key Words	*delegate*		
Rephrase			
Rule Out Choices			
A	B (X)	C	D (X)

not within scope of practice

HESI Test Question Approach

Positive?		YES	NO
Key Words			
Rephrase			
Rule Out Choices			
A (X)	B	C (X)	D

not appropriate

The charge nurse is making assignments for each of four staff members, including a registered nurse (RN), a practical nurse (PN), and two UAPs (UCPs). Which task is best assigned to the PN?

A. Maintain a 24-hour urine collection.
B. Wean a client from a mechanical ventilator.
C. Perform sterile wound irrigation.
D. Obtain scheduled vital signs.

HESI Test Question Approach			
Positive?		YES	NO
Key Words			
Rephrase			
Rule Out Choices			
~~A~~	~~B~~	C	~~D~~
UAP	RN only		UAP

Supervision Skills

- Direction/guidance
- Evaluation/monitoring
- Follow-up

Which situation warrants a variance (incident) report by the nurse?

A. A client refuses to take prescribed medication.
B. A client's status improves before completion of the course of medication.
C. A client has an allergic reaction to a prescribed medication.
D. A client received medication prescribed for another client.

HESI Test Question Approach			
Positive?		YES	NO
Key Words			
Rephrase			
Rule Out Choices			
~~A~~	~~B~~	~~C~~	D
document (why? Reeducate) & notify provider		Adverse drug rx report	

Handoff Communication

- A communication in which important client information is shared at pertinent points of care (e.g., change of shift, transfer from one clinical setting to another).
- Ensures continuity of care and client safety.
- Improves communication and appropriate delegation.

A nurse is preparing for change of shift. Which action by the nurse is characteristic of ineffective handoff communication?

A. The nurse states to the nurse coming on duty, "The client is anxious about his pain after surgery. Review the information I gave him about how to use an incentive spirometer."
B. The nurse refers to the electronic medical record (EMR) to review the client's medication administration record.
C. During rounds the nurse talks about the problem the UAP created by not performing a fingerstick blood glucose test on the client. *inappropriate*
D. Before giving report, the nurse performs rounds on her assigned clients so that there is less likelihood of interruption during handoff.

Continuity & delegation

HESI Test Question Approach			
Positive?		YES	(NO)
Key Words			
Rephrase			
Rule Out Choices			
A	B	C	D

S-BAR

S-BAR is an interdisciplinary communication strategy that promotes effective communication between caregivers.

S SITUATION—State the issue or problem.

B BACKGROUND—Provide the client's history.

A ASSESSMENT—Give the most recent vital signs and current findings.

R RECOMMENDATION—State what should be done.

The charge nurse is planning client assignments for the shift. The care team includes a registered nurse (RN), a practical nurse (PN), and unlicensed assistive personnel (UAP) (Unregulated Care Provider [UCP]) on the care team. Which client(s) could be assigned to the PN? (Select all that apply).

A. A client scheduled for a STAT x-ray scan after a fall on his hip.

B. A client receiving IV vancomycin (Vancocin) through a peripherally inserted central catheter (PICC) line.

C. A client with sickle cell crisis who was transferred from the ICU to the acute care area and who is receiving hydromorphone (Dilaudid) via a PCA pump. *too unstable*

D. A client with a pressure ulcer who was prescribed negative pressure (Wound VAC) care.

E. A postoperative client who has been prescribed 2 units of packed red blood cells.

role of RN

A charge nurse is making assignments for five clients. The nursing team has an RN, a PN, and two UAPs. Which client(s) would be assigned to the RN? (Select all that apply.)

A. A client from the previous shift with unstable angina.

B. A client with a stage 3 pressure ulcer who needs a bed bath.

C. A client with an enteral feeding absorbing at 30 mL/hour.

D. A cardiotomy client who is day 2 postoperative and who has chest tubes.

E. A client with quadriplegia for whom urinary catheterization has been prescribed.

HESI Test Question Approach			
Positive?		YES	NO
Key Words			
Rephrase			
depends on state (PICC line management)			
Rule Out Choices			
A	B	C	D

HESI Test Question Approach			
Positive?		YES	NO
Key Words			
Rephrase			
Rule Out Choices			
A	B	C	D

3 Clinical Concepts and Mechanisms of Disease

30 March 2016

Helen
Freeman → freeman44@msn.com

Pain

- Pain is whatever the client says it is.
- Pain occurs in all clinical settings.
- Nurses have a central role in pain assessment and management.
  - Assessing and reassessing pain and communicating with other healthcare providers
  - Ensuring the initiation and coordination of adequate pain relief measures
  - Evaluating the effectiveness of interventions
  - Advocating for clients with pain
- Pain medications generally are divided into three categories.
  - *Nonopioids* for mild pain or in combination for moderate pain
  - *Opioids* for moderate to severe pain
  - *Co-analgesic* or *adjuvant* drugs (i.e., anticonvulsants, antidepressants) for neuropathic pain

Types of Pain Medications
Nonopioid Analgesics Examples

- Acetaminophen (Tylenol)
  - Maximum recommended dosage is 4,000 mg (4 g) in 24 hours
  - Monitor liver function
- Salicylates
  - Aspirin
- Nonsteroidal antiinflammatory drugs (NSAIDs)
  - Ibuprofen (Motrin, Advil)
  - Indomethacin (Indocin)
  - Ketorolac (Toradol)
- Cyclooxygenase-2 (COX-2) inhibitors
  - Celecoxib (Celebrex)

NSAIDs (except aspirin) have been linked to a higher risk for increased cardiovascular events, such as myocardial infarction, stroke, and heart failure.

Clients who have just had heart surgery should not take NSAIDs.

Opioid Analgesics

- Mu agonists
  - Morphine sulfate (Doloral, Kadian, M-Eslon, MS Contin)
  - Hydromorphone (Dilaudid)
  - Meperidine hydrochloride (Demerol, Pethidine)
  - Methadone hydrochloride (Metadol)
  - Levorphanol (Levo-Dromoran)

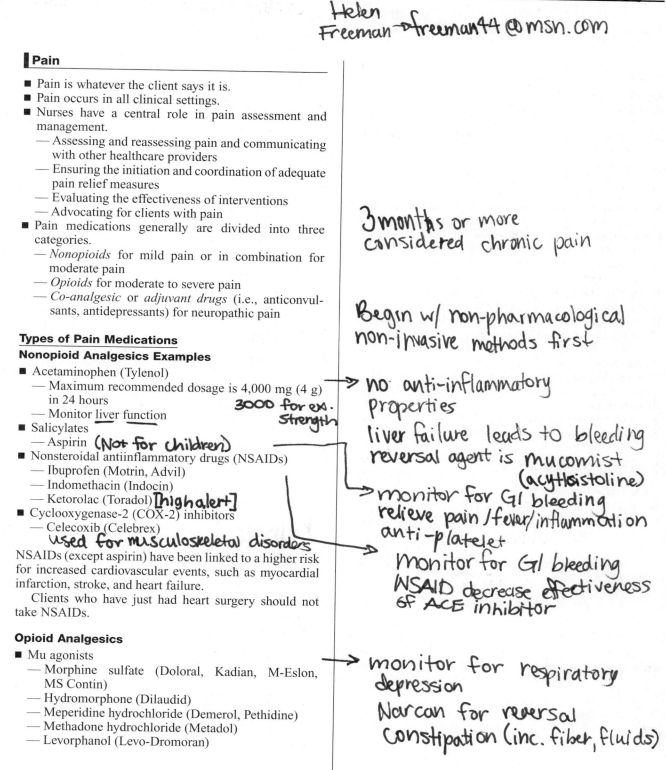

Handwritten annotations:

3 months or more considered chronic pain

Begin w/ non-pharmacological non-invasive methods first

3000 for ex. strength

(Not for children)

[high alert]

used for musculoskeletal disorders

no anti-inflammatory properties
liver failure leads to bleeding
reversal agent is mucomist (acytloistoline)

monitor for GI bleeding
relieve pain / fever / inflammation
anti-platelet
monitor for GI bleeding
NSAID decrease effectiveness of ACE inhibitor

monitor for respiratory depression
Narcan for reversal
Constipation (inc. fiber, fluids)

— Fentanyl (Duragesic)
— Oxycodone hydrochloride (Percocet, Percodan, Endocet, OxyContin, Oxy-IR, Supeudol)
— Hydrocodone (Lortab, Vicodin, Zydone)
— Codeine sulfate
■ Partial agonists
— Buprenorphine hydrochloride
— Butorphanol
— Nalbuphine hydrochloride (Nubain)
— Pentazocine hydrochloride (Talwin)
■ Adjuvant drugs
— Used for neuropathic pain
— Anticonvulsants, antidepressants, and anesthetics are prescribed alone or in combination with opioids for neuropathic pain
— Corticosteroids

[handwritten, right margin:] → combination agents no OTC acetominophen

[handwritten, right margin:] corticosteroids dec. inflammation

When opioids are prescribed for moderate pain, they are usually combined with a nonopioid analgesic, such as acetaminophen (e.g., codeine plus acetaminophen [Tylenol #3], hydrocodone plus acetaminophen [Vicodin]). Addition of acetaminophen or a NSAID limits the total daily dose that can be given.

Nonpharmacological Pain Relief Techniques

■ Noninvasive
— Heat and cold application
— Massage therapy
— Relaxation techniques
— Guided imagery
— Biofeedback techniques
■ Invasive
— Nerve blocks
— Interruption of neural pathways
— Acupuncture

[handwritten, right margin:] reposition breathing

Fluids and Electrolytes

Fluid Volume Excess

■ Causes
— CHF (most common), renal failure, cirrhosis, overhydration *(handwritten: (eldery, peds))*
■ Symptoms
— Peripheral edema, periorbital edema, elevated BP, dyspnea, altered LOC *(handwritten: ↓ JVD)*
■ Lab findings
— ↓ BUN, ↓ Hgb, ↓ Hct, ↓ serum osmolality, ↓ urine specific gravity
■ Treatment
—Diuretics, fluid restrictions, weigh daily, monitor K^+

[handwritten, right margin:] kidneys lungs aldosterone (sodium retention) ADH

[handwritten, bottom left:] loop, thiazide, spironolactone (K+ sparing) manage htn

A client is transferred to the intensive care unit immediately after a craniotomy on a ventilator. IVs hanging are a fentanyl PCA pump, D5N with 20 mEq KCl/L, and 1 unit of packed red blood cells with normal saline. The nurse reviews the MAR and finds that the client reports an allergy to fentanyl and sulfamethoxazole-trimethoprim (cotrimoxazole). What action should the nurse take first?

A. Auscultate lung sounds for wheezing.
B. Stop the fentanyl PCA pump.
C. Notify the healthcare provider immediately.
D. Contact the healthcare proxy to verify allergies.

HESI Test Question Approach			
Positive?		YES	NO
Key Words	allergies Fentanyl Fentanyl		
Rephrase			
Rule Out Choices			
A ✗	B	C	D

Fluid Volume Deficit

- Causes
  - Inadequate fluid intake, hemorrhage, vomiting, diarrhea, massive edema
- Symptoms
  - Weight loss, oliguria, postural hypotension, *skin turgor*
- Lab findings
  - $\uparrow$ BUN and $\uparrow$ or normal creatinine ($\uparrow$ Hgb, $\uparrow$ Hct, $\uparrow$ urine specific gravity
- Treatment
  - Strict I & O, replace with isotonic fluids, monitor BP, weigh daily

LR & NS

Electrolyte Balance

- Intracellular
  - K^+ maintains osmotic pressure.
  - K^+ imbalances may be life threatening.
- Extracellular
  - Na^+ maintains most abundant osmotic pressure.
  - REMEMBER: When either the ECF or the ICF changes in concentration, fluid shifts from the area of lesser concentration to the area of greater concentration.

135-145

Types of Imbalance

Hyponatremia

- Na^+ <135 mmol/L (mEq/L)
- Muscle cramps, confusion
- Check BP frequently
- Restrict fluids, cautious IV replacement as needed

Hypernatremia

- Na^+ >145 mmol/L (mEq/L)
- Pulmonary edema, seizures, thirst, fever
- No IVs that contain sodium
- Restrict sodium in diet
- Weigh daily

Hypokalemia

- K^+ <3.5 mmol/L (mEq/L)
- Rapid, thready pulse, flat T waves, fatigue, anorexia, muscle cramps
- IV potassium supplements
- Encourage foods high in K^+ (bananas, oranges, spinach)

milk & milk products

Brain needs Na^+ & glucose to function properly

Low Na^+ → seizures, give salt, processed foods

High Na^+ → pulmonary edema, seizures (crackles, dyspnea) give Lasix to dec. fluid in lungs

PO potassium (irritating to stomach)
IV K^+ (give slowly & diluted)

Hyperkalemia

- K$^+$ > 5.5 mmol/L (mEq/L)
- Tall, tented T waves, bradycardia, muscle weakness
- 10% to 20% glucose with regular insulin *insulin & D5W in emergency situations*
- Kayexalate → *causes excretion of K$^+$*
- Renal dialysis *→ pull off volume, Na$^+$, K$^+$, phosphate (Ca$^+$ ↑)*

Hypocalcemia

- Ca^{2+} <2.25 mmol/L (<9.0 mEq/L) *twitching of face*
- + Trousseau's sign, + Chvostek's sign, diarrhea, numbness, convulsions *carpal spasm*
- Administer calcium supplements
- IV calcium—give slowly
- Increase dietary calcium

Hypercalcemia

- Ca^{2+} >2.75 mmol/L (>10.5 mEq/L)
- Muscle weakness, constipation, nausea and vomiting (N/V), dysrhythmias, behavioral changes
- Limit vitamin D intake
- Avoid calcium-based antacids
- Administer calcitonin to reduce calcium
- Renal dialysis may be required

IV Therapy

- Types of IV fluids
  — *Isotonic:* 0.9% NS, LR, D$_5$W
  — *Hypotonic:* 0.5% NS, 0.45% NS → *osmolality lower than blood*
  — *Hypertonic:* D$_5$ 0.45% NS, D$_5$LR, D$_5$NS → *osmolality higher than blood*

Acid Base

The following are the basics for interpretation of ABG results on the NCLEX-RN Exam:

- pH
  — Normal = 7.35-7.45
  — <7.35 = acidosis
  — >7.45 = alkalosis
- pCO$_2$ *resp.*
  — Normal = 35-45 mmHg
  — >45 = acidosis
  — <35 = alkalosis
- HCO$_3^-$ *metabolic*
  — Normal = 21-28 mmol/L (21-28 mEq/L)
  — <21 = acidosis
  — >28 = alkalosis

Arterial Blood Gas Interpretation Practice →

Determine whether each set of ABGs indicates that the patient is normal, acidotic, or alkalotic. (Fill in the blank.)

1. pH = 7.32 ↓
   pCO$_2$ = 50 ↑
   HCO$_3^-$ = 25 –

This client is _____.

2. pH = 7.28 ↓
   pCO$_2$ = 35 –
   HCO$_3^-$ = 18 ↓

This client is _____.

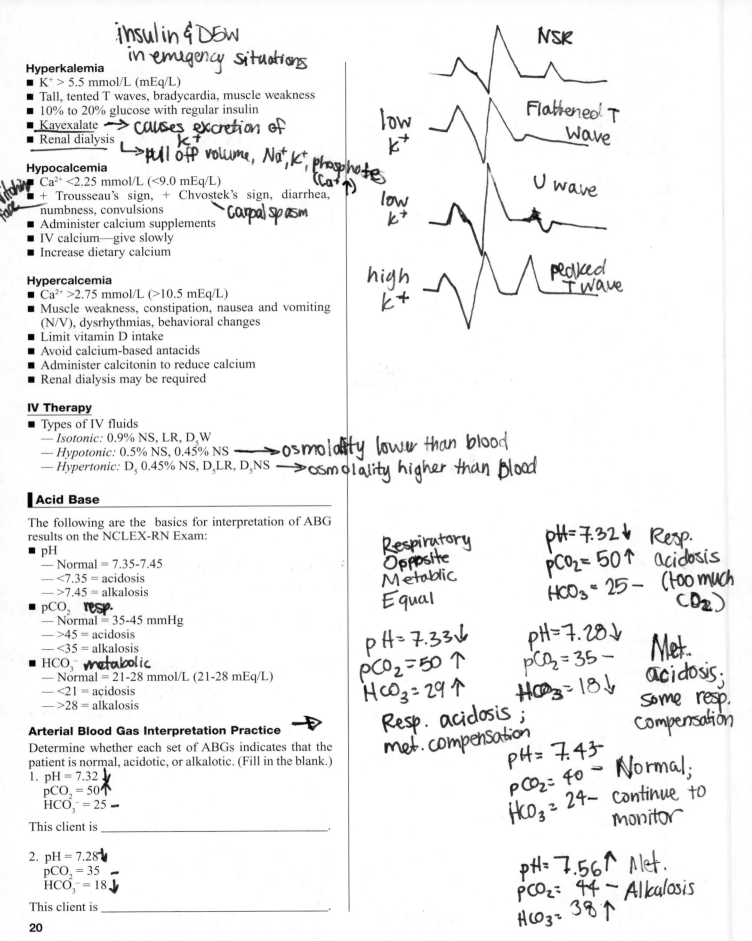

NSR

low K$^+$ — Flattened T wave

low K$^+$ — U wave

high K$^+$ — peaked T wave

Respiratory Opposite
Metabolic Equal

pH = 7.32 ↓ Resp.
pCO$_2$ = 50 ↑ acidosis
HCO$_3$ = 25 – (too much CO$_2$)

pH = 7.33 ↓
pCO$_2$ = 50 ↑
HCO$_3$ = 29 ↑
Resp. acidosis; met. compensation

pH = 7.28 ↓
pCO$_2$ = 35 –
HCO$_3$ = 18 ↓
Met. acidosis; some resp. compensation

pH = 7.43 –
pCO$_2$ = 40 –
HCO$_3$ = 24 –
Normal; continue to monitor

pH = 7.56 ↑ Met.
pCO$_2$ = 44 – Alkalosis
HCO$_3$ = 38 ↑

3. pH = 7.43 —
   pCO_2 = 40 —
   HCO_3^- = 24 —

This client is _____.

4. pH = 7.56 ↑
   pCO_2 = 44 —
   HCO_3^- = 38 ↑

This client is _____.

5. pH = 7.33 ↓
   pCO_2 = 50 ↑
   HCO_3^- = 29 ↑

This client is _____.

Safety

Falls
■ Sentinel event
■ Risk factors
— *Adult:* Stroke, depression, mobility issues, history of seizure, history of falls, use of assistive devices, polypharmacy, environmental issues, forgetting or ignoring mobility issues
— *Infants/children:* Length of stay, IV or saline lock, use of antiseizure medications, acute or chronic orthopedic diagnosis, receiving physical or occupational therapy, history of falling

Nursing and Collaborative Management
■ Fall prevention
— Safety surveillance
— Assess need for pain relief, toileting, positioning
— Frequent reorientation
— Client and family education
— Address environmental concerns
— Sitter

High-Alert Medications
■ High-alert medications are most likely to cause significant harm to the client even when used as intended.
■ Anticoagulants, narcotics and opiates, insulin, chemotherapeutic drugs, and sedatives are the most common high-alert medications.
■ The most common types of harm associated with these medications are hypotension, bleeding, hypoglycemia, delirium, lethargy, and bradycardia.
■ Strategies to prevent harm
— Built-in redundancies
— Double-checking
— Smart pumps
— Standardized or protocol order sets

A client is receiving an infusion of dobutamine hydrochloride. The order reads: Infuse dobutamine IV at 5 mcg/kg/min. 500 mg in 250 mL D_5W. The client weighs 65 kg. Calculate the flow rate in mL/hr.

The flow rate is __**9.75**__ mL/hr.

Death and Grief

- Stages of grief
  — Denial
  — Anger
  — Bargaining
  — Depression
  — Acceptance
- Encourage the client to express anger.
- Do not take away the defense mechanism or coping mechanism the client uses in a crisis.
- Customs surrounding death and dying vary among cultures. The nurse must make every attempt to understand and accommodate the family's cultural traditions when caring for a dying client.

Infection and HIV

Infection

- Invasion of the body by a pathogen
- Response to the invasion
  — Localized
  — Systemic
- Nosocomial infections
  — Acquired as a result of exposure to a microorganism in a hospital setting

Human Immunodeficiency Virus
Routes of Transmission

- Unprotected sexual contact
  — Most common mode of transmission
- Exposure to blood through drug-using equipment
- Perinatal transmission
  — Most common route of infection for children
- Can occur during pregnancy, at the time of delivery, or after birth through breast-feeding

Nursing Assessment

- Laboratory testing
- Positive result on enzyme immunoassay (EIA) formally enzyme-linked immunosorbent assay (ELISA)
- Confirmed with Western blot test
- Polymerase chain reaction (PCR) (*used with neonate)
- OraQuick In-Home HIV Test: Positive result is only preliminary; it must be confirmed by a healthcare professional.

0.325 mg/min
19.5 mg/hr

$$\frac{19.5 mg}{? mL} = \frac{500 mg}{250 mL}$$

9.75 mL

Symptoms
- May begin with flulike symptoms in the earliest stage and advance to …
  — Severe weight loss
  — Secondary infections
  — Cancers
  — Neurological disease

Nursing and Collaborative Management
- Monitor disease progression and immune function
- Initiate and monitor antiretroviral therapy (ART)
- Prevent development of opportunistic diseases
- Detect and treat opportunistic diseases
- Manage symptoms
- Prevent or decrease complications of treatment
- Prevent transmission of HIV

Ongoing assessment, interaction with the client, and client education and support are required to accomplish these objectives.

HIV Drug Therapy
The goals of drug therapy are to:
- Reduce the viral load
- Maintain or raise the CD4+ T-cell counts
- Delay the development of HIV-related symptoms and opportunistic diseases

Nursing and Collaborative Management
- The client should have regular blood counts to track CD4 levels and the viral load.
- Side effects are common, and there are many drug-drug interactions.

HIV Medications
- Nucleoside reverse transcriptase inhibitors (NRTIs)
  — Zidovudine (AZT) Retrovir) *only drug used in pregnancy*
  — Lamivudine (3TC, Epivir-HBV, Heptovir)
  — Abacavir sulfate (Ziagen)
  — Emtricitabine (Emtriva)
  — Tenofovir disoproxil (Viread)

Non-nucleoside reverse transcriptase inhibitors (NNRTIs)
- NNRTI's are able to convert into enzymes that inhibit viral replication. A serious, harmful side effect is hepatotoxicity. → *Reduces contraceptive effects*
- Enzymes, hepatotoxicity
  — Nevirapine (Viramune)
  — Delavirdine mesylate (Rescriptor)
  — Efavirenz (Sustiva)
- Protease inhibitors (PIs) → *Avoid high fat/ high protein foods*
  — Indinavir sulfate (Crixivan)
  — Ritonavir (Norvir)
  — Nelfinavir mesylate (Viracept)
  — Atazanavir (Reyataz)
  — Fosamprenavir (Telzir)
- Entry inhibitor
  — Enfuvirtide (Fuzeon)

Pt. must take exactly as prescribed

Monitor for lactic acidosis liver function

Safety in med. administration

Pediatric HIV

Common clinical manifestations of HIV infection in children include:

- Lymphadenopathy
- Hepatosplenomegaly
- Oral candidiasis
- Chronic or recurrent diarrhea
- Failure to thrive *(dec. appetite)*
- Developmental delay
- Parotitis

Considerations

- Client education concerns transmission and control of infectious diseases.
- Safety issues include appropriate storage of special medications and equipment.
- Prevention is a key component of HIV education.
- Aggressive pain management is essential.
- Common psychosocial concerns include disclosure of the diagnosis.
- ✱ If an HIV-infected mother is treated with zidovudine during pregnancy and the neonate is treated after birth, the probability of HIV infection of the child decreases from 30% to 4% to 8%.
- Avoid exposure to individuals with infections (e.g., chickenpox).
- Administer no live viruses.

Avoid exposure to chicken pox
No live vaccination

Cancer

Leukemia

- Acute myelogenous leukemia (AML)
  - Inability of leukocytes to mature; those that do are abnormal
  - Clients usually 60 to 70 years of age
  - Poor prognosis *IV chemo*
- Chronic myelogenous leukemia (CML)
  - Abnormal production of granulocytic cells
  - Clients usually 20 to 60 years of age (peak is about age 45)
  - Poor prognosis *Oral chemo*
- Acute lymphocytic leukemia (ALL)
  - Abnormal leukocytes in blood-forming tissue
  - Usually seen before 14 years of age and in older adults
  - Favorable prognosis *IV chemo*
- Chronic lymphocytic leukemia (CLL)
  - Increased production of leukocytes and lymphocytes in the bone marrow, spleen, and liver
  - Clients usually 50 to 70 years of age
  - 5-year survival rate: 73% overall

Cancer of blood forming organs

Leukopenia
Immunosuppression
Thrombocytopenia
Anemia (↓ H&H)

Bone Marrow biopsy
Biphasic
Acute phase followed by chronic slow-progressing
*   coorelated w/ Philadelphia chromosome)*

Pt. may be asymptomatic slow-progressing

Nursing Assessment

- General
  - Fever, generalized lymphadenopathy, lethargy, epistaxis
- Integumentary
  - Pallor or jaundice; petechiae, ecchymoses, purpura, reddish brown to purple cutaneous infiltrates, macules, and papules

- Cardiovascular
  — Tachycardia, systolic murmurs
- Gastrointestinal
  — Gingival bleeding and hyperplasia; oral ulcerations, herpes, and *Candida* infections; perirectal irritation and infection; hepatomegaly, splenomegaly
- Neurological
  — Seizures, disorientation, confusion, decreased coordination, cranial nerve palsies, papilledema
- Musculoskeletal
  — Muscle wasting, bone pain, joint pain

Medications for Leukemia
- Alkylating agents
- Antimetabolites → *methotrexate (very toxic to body)*
- Corticosteroids
- Nitrosoureas
- Mitotic inhibitors/vinca alkaloids
- Biological therapy
- Epipodophyllotoxin derivatives
- Retinoid

drugs:
Chemo vesicant- can cause extravasation
(Also cipro, dopamine, etc.)
check for patency of line
concurrent lucovorin rescue

Nursing and Collaborative Management for Clients with Immunodeficiency and/or Bone Marrow Suppression
- Monitor WBC count
- Report fever or S/S of infection to physician as soon as symptoms are recognized
- Teach infection control measures
- Administer IV antibiotics as ordered:
  — Trough (draw shortly before administration)
  — Peak (30 minutes to 1 hour after administration)

Hodgkin's Lymphoma
Etiology
- Epstein-Barr virus (EBV), genetic predisposition, and exposure to occupational toxins

most often found in young white males

Diagnosis
- The main diagnostic feature of Hodgkin's lymphoma is the presence of Reed-Sternberg cells in lymph node biopsy specimens.

Nursing Assessment
- Weight loss
- Fatigue
- Weakness
- Chills, fever, night sweats
- Tachycardia

lymph node enlargement

Nursing and Collaborative Management
- Chemotherapy
- Radiation therapy
- Pain management due to tumors
- Pancytopenia
- Fertility
- Secondary malignancies

Monitor for spleen/liver involvement

IV chemo, external beam radiation

→ Treatment may lead to infertility

Non-Hodgkin's Lymphoma

Etiology
- Immunosuppressant medications, age, and HIV, EBV infection
- Affects the beta or T cells

Diagnosis
- Biopsy
- MRI, CT scan

Nursing Assessment
- Painless lymph node enlargement (lymphadenopathy)
- Depending on where the disease has spread, same as for Hodgkin's lymphoma

Treatment
- Chemotherapy (sometimes radiation therapy)
- Monoclonal antibodies
- Symptom management (depending on affected system)

Nursing and Collaborative Management
- Strict aseptic technique
- Protect client from infection
- Monitor for S/S of anemia
- High-nutrient diet
- Emotional support for client and family
- Treatment must be completed to help ensure client's survival.
  — Highly curable disease when diagnosed early and treatment is completed

slow-progressing

A client is receiving vancomycin (Vancocin) IV and has a prescription for peak and trough levels. Before administering the next dose, what action should the nurse take?
A. Verify the culture and sensitivity results.
B. Review the client's WBC count.
C. Schedule the collection of blood for a peak level.
D. Determine whether the trough level has been collected.

HESI Test Question Approach		
Positive?	YES	NO
Key Words	*peak & trough levels*	
	action	
Rephrase		
Rule Out Choices		
A	X	X	D

not important right now

Administration of Chemotherapeutic Agents
- Strict guidelines must be followed!
- These drugs normally are administered by a chemotherapy-certified RN.
- Pregnant nurses should not administer most of these agents.
- Wear Personal Protective Equipment (PPE) for hazardous drug handling.
  — Gowns – disposable, made of fabric that has low-permeability to the agents in use, with closed-front and cuffs, intended for single use.

— Gloves – powder-free, labeled and tested for use with chemotherapy drugs, made of latex, nitrile, or neoprene.
— Face and eye protection when splashing is possible.
— An approved respirator when there is a risk of inhaling drug aerosols (such as during spill or clean up).
- Types of IV catheters:
— Hickman
— Broviac
— Port-a-cath

The CBC results for a client receiving chemotherapy are: hemoglobin–85 mmol/L (8.5 g/dL), hematocrit–32%, WBC count–6.5 × 10⁹/L (6,500 cells/mm³). Which meal choice is best for this client?
A. Grilled chicken, rice, fresh fruit salad, milk
B. Broiled steak, whole wheat rolls, spinach salad, coffee
C. Smoked ham, mashed potatoes, applesauce, iced tea
D. Tuna noodle casserole, garden salad, lemonade

[handwritten note: WBC ↓ 2000 is of concern. 2000]

HESI Test Question Approach		
Positive?	YES	NO
Key Words	*low Hgb* *low Normal Hct* *Normal WBC*	
Rephrase		
Rule Out Choices		
A	B	C	D

Head and Neck Cancer
- Typically squamous cell in origin
- Tumor sites
— Paranasal sinuses
— Oral cavity
— Nasopharynx
— Oropharynx
— Larynx
- Significant disability because of the potential loss of voice, disfigurement, and social consequences.
- Head and neck cancer is most common in males over age 50 and is related to heavy tobacco and alcohol intake.

Lung Cancer
- One of the leading causes of cancer-related deaths in Canada and US.
- The increase in death rates for both men and women is directly related to cigarette smoking.

Nursing Assessment
- Symptoms of lung cancer are not usually apparent until the disease is in the advanced stages.
- Persistent hacking cough may be either dry or productive with blood-tinged sputum.
- Hoarseness
- Dyspnea
- Abnormal chest radiograph
- Positive sputum on cytological examination

[handwritten note: typically not discovered early — cough — bloody sputum]

Treatment

- Chemotherapy
- Radiation therapy
- Surgical intervention
  — Pneumonectomy—removal of entire lung
  — Lobectomy—or segmental resection
- Nursing care depends on the type of medical treatment prescribed.

Immediate Postoperative Care

- Promote ventilation and re-expansion of the lung
  — Maintain a clear airway
  — Maintain the closed drainage system, if used
- Promote arm exercises to maintain full use on the operative side
- Promote good nutrition
- Monitor incision for bleeding and subcutaneous emphysema

May return w/ chest tube in place.

small amount of subcut emphysema is expected; mark extent

Colorectal Cancer

- The third most common form of cancer and the second leading cause of cancer-related deaths in the US and Canada.
  — Adenocarcinoma most common
  — Common metastasis to the liver

typically
Not discovered early

Symptoms

- Rectal bleeding
- Change in bowel habits
- Abdominal pain, weight loss, N/V
- Ribbonlike stool
- Sensation of incomplete evacuation

Diagnostic Testing

- Testing of stool for occult blood
- Colonoscopy

Treatment Modalities

- Chemotherapy
- Radiation therapy
- Adjunctive or palliative

Surgical Intervention

- Bowel resection
- Temporary colostomy
- Permanent colostomy

Postoperative Care Issues

- Stoma care
  — Loop
  — Double-barrel
  — End stoma
- Incision care
  — Abdominal
  — Perineal
- Packing and drains
  — HemoVac
  — Jackson-Pratt

Stoma Assessment

- Stoma should be pink. *, moist*
- Mild to moderate swelling of the stoma is normal for the first 2 to 3 weeks after surgery.
- Pouching system
  — Skin barrier
  — Bag or pouch
  — Adhesive
- Help client cope with the stoma.
  — Provide information
  — Teach practical stoma care techniques
- Help client address issues involving social interactions.
  — Employment
  — Body image
  — Sexuality

Call Dr. immediated for dark, dusky stoma

Teaching post-op & pre-op about care of a colostomy

The nurse is caring for a client who is 24-hours post procedure for a hemicolectomy with temporary colostomy placement. The nurse assesses the client's stoma, which is dry and dark red. What action should the nurse take based on this finding?

ischemia

A. Notify the healthcare provider of the finding.
B. Document the finding in the client's record.
C. Replace the pouch system over the stoma.
D. Place a petrolatum gauze dressing on the stoma.

HESI Test Question Approach		
Positive?	YES	NO
Key Words	*dry, dark red stoma action*	
Rephrase		
Rule Out Choices		
A	B	C	D

Abnormal finding

Breast Cancer

- Risks
  — Family history
  — Age
  — Hyperestrogenism
  — Radiation exposure
- Most tumors are discovered through breast self-examination. → *dimpling, immovable tumor, painless*
- Mammogram, ultrasound, MRI, biopsy
- Tumors tend to be located in the upper outer quadrant.
  — Ductal carcinoma
  — Lobar carcinoma
  — Ductal carcinoma in situ
  — Inflammatory breast cancer (most aggressive)
  — Paget's disease (areola and nipple)
- Recommend a mammogram every 1 to 2 years after age 40 and annually after age 50.

Treatment Modalities

- Surgical
  — Mastectomy
  — Modified radical mastectomy
  — Lumpectomy
  — Tissue expansion and breast implant
  — Musculocutaneous flap procedure
- Radiation
- Chemotherapy

Avoid IV & BP on sides of mastectomy

- Hormonal therapy
  — Tamoxifen (Nolvadex)—blocks estrogen receptors
  — Fulvestrant (Faslodex)—destroys estrogen receptors
  — Anastrozole (Arimidex), letrozole (Femara)—prevent production of estrogen
- Biological-targeted therapies
- Monoclonal antibodies

Nursing Assessment

- Hard lump, not freely moveable
- Dimpling in the skin
- Change in skin color
- Confirmed by mammogram and biopsy with frozen sections

Nursing Interventions

- Preoperative
  — Assess expectations
- Postoperative
  — Monitor for bleeding
  — Position arm on operative side on a pillow
  — No BP cuffs, IVs, or injections on operative side
  — Provide emotional support; recognize the grieving process

Cancer of the Cervix

- Human papillomavirus (HPV) infects the skin and mucous membranes of humans.
  — A vaccine (Gardasil) is available that reduces the incidence of both cervically related neoplasia and cervical cancer due to infection with HPV types 16 and 18. Only Gardasil is available for males and teenage boys and young men through age 21. The vaccine has been approved for females ages 9 to 26 and for teenage boys through age 21 (Gardasil).
  — The vaccination protocol requires three shots given over 6 months.
- Cervical cancer usually can be detected early with a Pap test.
- Dysplasia is treated with cryosurgery, laser treatment, conization, and possibly hysterectomy.
- Early carcinoma is treated with hysterectomy or intracavitary irradiation.
- Late carcinoma is treated with irradiation, chemotherapy, and/or pelvic exenteration.

[handwritten margin note: Pap Smear ages 21-70 even w/ hysterectomy]

Care of the Client with Radiation Implants

- Client is *not* radioactive
- Implants do contain radioactivity
- Place client in private room
- No pregnant caretakers or pregnant visitors
- Keep lead-lined container in room
- All of client's secretions may be radioactive
- Wear radiation badge when providing care

Ovarian Cancer

- Leading cause of death from gynecological cancer
- Greatest risk factor is family history
- Asymptomatic in early stages
- Generalized feeling of abdominal fullness
- Sense of pelvic heaviness
- Loss of appetite
- Change in bowel habits
- Late-stage symptoms
  — Pelvic discomfort
  — Low back pain
  — Abdominal pain

Testicular Cancer

- Feeling of heaviness in lower abdomen
- Painless lump/swelling
- Postoperative orchiectomy
- Observe for bleeding
- Encourage genetic counseling (sperm banking)

Self-checks every month
Good prognosis w/ early diagnosis

Postoperative Management

- Monitor for urine leaks
- Avoid rectal manipulation
- Low-residue diet *(to slow activity in GI tract)*

Cancer of the Prostate

- Symptoms of urinary obstruction
- Elevated prostate-specific antigen (PSA)
- Surgical removal of the prostate
- Follow-up radiation therapy and chemotherapy

monitor for bowel & bladder incotinence /impotence
No children around pt. w/ radiation seeds

The charge nurse is assigning rooms for four new clients. Only one private room is available on the oncology unit. Which client should be placed in the private room?

A. The client with ovarian cancer who is receiving chemotherapy.

B. The client with breast cancer who is receiving external beam irradiation.

C. The client with prostate cancer who has just had a transurethral resection.

D. The client with cervical cancer who is receiving intracavitary irradiation.

HESI Test Question Approach		
Positive?	YES	NO
Key Words	*private room*	
	radiation	
Rephrase		
Rule Out Choices		
~~A~~	B	~~C~~	D

Brain Tumor

- Primary malignant tumors can arise in any area of brain tissue.
- Benign tumors can continue to grow and cause problems with ↑ ICP.
- Assess for headache, vomiting, seizures, aphasia, and abnormal findings on CT, MRI, or PET scan.

Nursing and Collaborative Management

- Management is similar to that of a client with a head injury.
- Major concern is ↑ ICP.
- Keep HOB elevated 30 to 40 degrees.
- Radiation therapy
- Chemotherapy
- Surgical removal—craniotomy

Early signs include headache, vomiting (morning) (no nausea)
CSF drainage from nose & ear
- Meningitis risk

Postoperative Care

- Monitor for:
  - — ↑ ICP
  - — CSF leakage
- Monitor respiratory status closely.
- Monitor for seizure activity.

After the change of shift report, the nurse reviews her assignments. Which client should the RN assess first?

A. The elderly client receiving palliative care for heart failure who complains of constipation and nervousness.

(B) The adult client who is 48 hours postoperative for a colectomy and who is reported to be having nausea.

C. The middle-aged client with chronic renal failure whose urinary catheter has been draining 95 mL for 8 hours.

D. The client who is 2 days postoperative for a thoracotomy and who has chest tubes, is on oxygen at 3 L/min, and has a respiratory rate of 12 breaths/min.

Perioperative Care
Preoperative Care

- Preoperative evaluation
  - — Obtain a complete history, including:
    - List of current medications and allergies
    - Previous surgical experiences (response to anesthetic)
    - Signed consent
  - — Make sure informed consent has been obtained before client is sedated
  - — Preoperative teaching
    - NPO after midnight before surgery
    - Teach coughing and deep breathing, incentive spirometry
    - Review methods of pain control

Intraoperative Care

- Maintain the client's safety
  - — Surgical Care Improvement Project (SCIP) core measures are mandatory for client safety.
    - Emphasis is on preventing infection, serious cardiac events, and venous thromboembolism (VTE)
    - *Examples:* Administration of a prophylactic antibiotic within 1 hour of incision; glucose level <11.1 mmol/L (<200 mg/dL); removal of urinary catheter on postoperative day 1 (POD #1) or POD #2; maintenance of β- blocker therapy; provision of VTE prophylaxis
    - Mandatory time out
      - □ Confirm client's identity and consent, procedure to be performed, and surgical site
- Provide psychosocial support

HESI Test Question Approach		
Positive?	YES	NO
Key Words		
Rephrase		
Rule Out Choices		

no immediate needs

Postoperative Care

- Monitor for S/S of shock
- Position client on side → *prevent aspiration*
- Manage pain

One of the primary goals of postoperative care is to prevent common complications.

- Urinary retention
  — Check for bladder distention
- UTI
  — Removal of urinary catheter POD #1 or POD #2
- Pulmonary problems
  — Check breath sounds
  — Check O_2 saturation
- Decreased peristalsis
- Paralytic ileus
- Absent bowel sounds
- Wound dehiscence
- Wound evisceration
- VTE

ABCs
hemodynamic stability

Check for return of bowel sounds.
Mobility!
↳ prevents thromboembolism

Which laboratory result for a preoperative client would prompt the nurse to contact the healthcare provider?
A. Platelet count: 151×10^9/L (151,000/mm³) *[150,000 – 400,000]*
B. WBC count: 85 × 10⁹/L (8,500/mm³)
C. Serum potassium level: 2.8 mmol/L (mEq/L)
D. Urine specific gravity: 1.031

HESI Test Question Approach		
Positive?	YES	NO
Key Words		
Rephrase		
Rule Out Choices		
A	B ✗	C D ✗

normal values

A PN is assigned to care for an 82-year-old client who had a total right hip replacement with cement 2 days ago. Which observation(s) should the PN immediately report to the RN? (Select all that apply.)
A. The client complains of incisional pain, rating it a 6 on a scale of 0 to 10. *Ongoing*
B. The client has had a change in orientation to person but not to time or place.
C. Swelling and redness have developed in the client's lower left leg.
D. The PN emptied 15 mL of bloody drainage from the Jackson Pratt.
E. The client's last set of vital signs was: T–100.2° F, P–87, R–12, BP–108/74, O2 sat–93%.

Temperature not a reliable indicator of fever in older adults

HESI Test Question Approach		
Positive?	YES	NO
Key Words		
Rephrase		
Rule Out Choices		
A	B	C ✗ D

normal finding

The nurse is the first responder at the scene of a mass casualty incident. The nurse is tasked to triage the victims from highest to lowest priority. Please arrange the victims from highest to lowest priority. All options must be used.

5 A. Victim A is an elder adult with agonal respirations with open head injury

1 B. Victim B is a confused adult with bright red blood pulsating from a leg wound

3 C. Victim C is a young adult with multiple compound fractures of the arms and legs

2 D. Victim D is an adult with multiple shrapnel wounds of the face and arms complaining of abdominal pain

4 E. Victim E is a sobbing adult with several minor lacerations on the face, arms, and legs

HESI Test Question Approach		
Positive?	**YES**	**NO**
Key Words		
Rephrase		
Rule Out Choices		
A	B	C	D

The nurse is monitoring the status of a client recovering from a myocardial infarction. The nurse would become most concerned with which signs that could indicate an evolving problem?

A. A steady pulse of 88 beats/min
B. Rising systolic pressure from 110 to 120 mmHg
C. Six premature ventricular contractions/min
D. Total urine output of 110 ml/h over 3 hours

30 mL/hr is normal

HESI Test Question Approach		
Positive?	**YES**	**NO**
Key Words		
Rephrase		
Rule Out Choices		
~~A~~	~~B~~	C	~~D~~

normal range

Advanced Clinical Concepts

Shock
Stages of Shock

■ Stage 1: Initial
 — Early signs include agitation
 — Restlessness
 — ↑ Heart rate
 — Cool, pale skin
■ Stage 2: Compensatory
 — Cardiac output < 4-6 L/min
 — BP systolic < 100 mmHg
 — ↓ Urinary output
 — Confusion
 — Cerebral perfusion < 70 mmHg
■ Stage 3: Progressive
 — Edema
 — Excessively low BP
 — Dysrhythmia
 — Weak, thready pulses

Red - immediate, critical
Yellow - injured, can wait 30 min.
Green - Walking wounded
Black - dead, expected

SHOCK:
Widespread underperfusion of tissue & organs

Brain, heart, lungs most vital in terms of perfusion

- Stage 4: Irreversible
  — Profound hypotension
  — Unresponsive to vasopressors
  — Slowing heart rate
  — Multiple organ failure
  — Severe hypoxemia

Most likely leads to death

Types of Shock
- Hypovolemic
  — Most common
  — Related to internal or external blood/fluid loss
- Cardiogenic
  — Pump failure
  — Results in ↓ cardiac output
- Vasogenic (anaphylactic, neurogenic, and septic shock)
  — Excessive vasodilation and impaired distribution of blood flow
  — Failure of arteriolar resistance

Prevent loss of volume

Treatment for Shock
- Correct decreased tissue perfusion and restore cardiac output
  — Optimize oxygenation and ventilation
  — Fluid resuscitation
    - Cause of shock dictates type of treatment
    - Volume expanders for hypovolemia *; Isotonic fluids*
    - Cardiogenic shock: Volume expanders may precipitate pulmonary edema
  — Drug therapy
    - Restoration of cardiac function is based on the effect of shock on preload, afterload, and contractility
      □ Preload
        ◆ Increase preload through colloids or crystalloids
        ◆ Decrease preload through nitrates, diuretics, or morphine
      □ Afterload
        ◆ Increase afterload through pressors
        ◆ Decrease afterload through nitroprusside (Nipride), ACE-I, or ARBs → *easier to control BP*
      □ Contractility
        ◆ Increase contractility through dobutamine, digoxin (Lanoxin)
        ◆ Decrease contractility through β-blockers, calcium channel blockers

MAP = $\dfrac{\text{systolic} + 2(\text{diastolic})}{3}$

Should be ⩾ 70

A client in shock develops a mean arterial pressure (MAP) of 60 mmHg and a heart rate of 110 beats/min. Which prescribed intervention should the nurse implement first?
A. Increase the rate of O_2 flow.
B. Obtain arterial blood gas results.
C. Insert an indwelling urinary catheter.
D. Increase the rate of IV fluids.

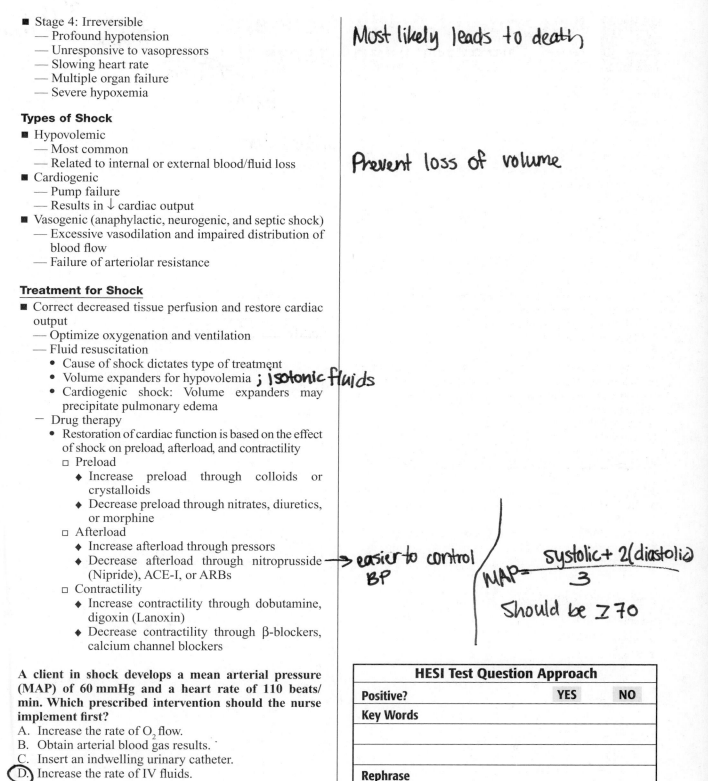

HESI Test Question Approach		
Positive?	YES	NO
Key Words		
Rephrase		
Rule Out Choices		
A	B	C	D

Chapter **4** **Advanced Clinical Concepts and Disaster Management**

Cascade of Sepsis

Septic shock is one component of the systemic inflammatory response syndrome (SIRS). The syndrome starts with an infection, which progresses to *bacteremia,* then *sepsis,* then *severe sepsis,* then *septic shock,* and finally to multiple organ dysfunction syndrome (MODS).

Systemic inflammatory response syndrome (SIRS) is a systemic inflammatory response to an assortment of insults, including sepsis, ischemia, infarction, and injury. Generalized inflammation in organs remote from the initial insult characterizes the syndrome.

Multiple organ dysfunction syndrome (MODS) is the failure of two or more organ systems in an acutely ill client such that homeostasis cannot be maintained without intervention. MODS results from SIRS. These two syndromes represent the two ends of a continuum.

Nursing and Collaborative Management

- Prevention strategies
- Early screening for subtle changes in HR, systolic pressure, respiratory rate, oxygen saturation, urinary output, and central nervous system changes
- Lactic acid blood levels
- Prevention and treatment of infection
  - Blood culture before starting antibiotics
  - Broad-spectrum antibiotics within 1 to 3 hours of admission
  - Maintenance of tissue oxygenation
  - Nutritional and metabolic support
  - Support of individual failing organs

Disseminated Intravascular Coagulation (DIC)

DIC is an abnormal response of the normal clotting cascade; it is stimulated by a disease process or disorder.

- DIC results from abnormally initiated and accelerated clotting.
- A decrease in clotting factors and platelets ensues.
- This decrease may lead to uncontrollable hemorrhage.
- As more clots are made, more breakdown products from fibrinogen and fibrin are also formed. They interfere with blood coagulation in three ways, by:
  - Coating the platelets and interfering with platelet function
  - Interfering with thrombin, thereby disrupting coagulation
  - Attaching to fibrinogen, thus interfering with the process necessary to form a clot
- ↑D-Dimer assay test measuring the degree of fibrinolysis and ↑ Fibrin Split Products.
- Appropriate nursing interventions are essential to the client's survival.
- Astute, ongoing assessment is required.
  - Early detection of bleeding, both occult and overt, must be a primary goal.
    - Assess the client for signs of external and internal bleeding.
  - Be alert for manifestations of the syndrome.

Bacteremia → Sepsis → Severe Sepsis → Septic Shock → MODS (2 or more organs)

Lactic Acid monitoring

- Institution of appropriate treatment measures, which can be challenging and sometimes paradoxic
  — Heparin infusion
  — Blood and FFP transfusions and cryoprecipitate

Acute Respiratory Distress Syndrome (ARDS)

- ARDS is considered to be present if the client has the following:
  — Refractory hypoxemia
  — New bilateral interstitial or alveolar infiltrates on a chest radiograph (this condition on a radiographic study is often called "whiteout or" "white lung")
  — Pulmonary artery wedge pressure of 18 mmHg or less and no evidence of heart failure
  — A predisposing condition for ARDS within 48 hours of clinical manifestations
  — Alveolar capillary membrane damage with subsequent leakage of fluids into the interstitial spaces and the alveoli
- As ARDS progresses, it is associated with profound respiratory distress requiring endotracheal intubation and PPV.

Nursing Assessment

- Dyspnea
- Scattered crackles
- Intercostal retractions
- Pink frothy sputum
- Cyanosis
- Hypoxemia
- Hypercapnia
- Respiratory acidosis
  — Impaired gas exchange
- Increased secretions
- Decreased cardiac output

Lung fields whited-out on x-ray due to fluid

Nursing and Collaborative Management

- Overall goals for a client with ARDS
  — Pao_2 of at least 60 mmHg
  — Adequate lung ventilation to maintain normal pH
- Goals for a client recovering from ARDS
  — Pao_2 within normal limits for age or baseline values on room air
  — $Sao_2 > 90\%$
  — Patent airway
  — Clear lungs on auscultation
- Positive end-expiratory pressure (PEEP) $\longrightarrow$ *holds alveoli open to allow for better gas exchange*
  — A ventilatory option that creates positive pressure at end exhalation and restores functional residual capacity (FRC)

Delirium

- An acute state of confusion, commonly occurring in the elderly, that may indicate an impending change in condition
- Risk factors
  — Use of opioids and/or corticosteroids
  — Drug or alcohol abuse

- UTI, fluid and electrolyte imbalance
- Postoperative, ICU, or emergent delirium
- Sleep deprivation, advanced age or vision, and hearing impairment

Nursing and Collaborative Management

- Monitor neurological status on an ongoing basis
- Provide a low-stimulation environment
- Approach the client slowly and from the front
- Provide the appropriate level of supervision/surveillance
- Reorient the client and communicate with simple statements
- Consider management with neuroleptic drugs (e.g., haloperidol)
- Encourage family visibility and support

Life Support

- Cardiac arrest is the most common event requiring CPR.
- C-A-B—*C*hest compressions–*A*irway–*B*reathing
  - Emphasis is on high-quality chest compressions
  - Push hard and push fast
  - Adult 100 compressions/min
- In-hospital cardiac arrest
  - Initiate CPR with BCLS guidelines, moving to advanced cardiac life support (ACLS) guidelines
  - Determine unresponsiveness
  - Activate emergency response or cardiac arrest team
  - Obtain AED and/or emergency crash cart (do not leave client)
  - If pulse is not identified with 10 seconds:
    - Establish an airway
    - Ventilate with 2 breaths via manual resuscitation (breathing) bag (e.g., Ambu)
    - Maintain compressions-to-breaths ratio of 30:2
    - Apply quick look paddles or AED to determine whether defibrillation is necessary; defibrillate as indicated, following hospital policies and procedures
    - Prepare to administer epinephrine if indicated

CPR and Choking Basics: Neonates and Children 1 to 8 Years

- Most common indications for CPR in children are not the same as those for adults.
  - *Neonates and infants:* Hypoxia, hypoglycemia, hypothermia, acidosis, hypercoagulability
  - *Children:* Respiratory arrest, prolonged hypoxemia secondary to respiratory insult or shock, including septic shock
- Guidelines vary based on child's age.
  - If no response occurs, call a "code," or cardiac arrest, to initiate response of cardiac arrest team. Obtain AED or emergency crash cart with defibrillator.
  - Check for pulse.
    - *Infant < 1 year:* Brachial pulse
    - *Children 1 year to puberty:* Carotid or femoral

— Compressions
- *Infants (most):* Compressions are applied over at least one third of the anterior/posterior diameter of the chest to a depth of 1½ inches.
- *Children (most):* Compressions are applied over at least one third of the anterior/posterior diameter of the chest to a depth of 2 inches.
- One rescuer: 30 compressions to 2 breaths; two rescuers:15 compressions to 1 breath
- Deliver each breath over 1 second (avoid excess ventilation (gastric inflation)

For up-to-date information on FBOA and CPR, see the American Heart Association website for CPR guidelines: *www.heart.org/HEARTORG/.*

Disaster Management

- The nurse is an active team member in the event of biological, chemical, radioactive, mass trauma, and natural disasters.
- The nurse plays a role at all three levels of disaster management.

Preparedness...Response...Recovery
- Levels of prevention in disaster management
  - *Primary:* Planning, training, educating personnel and the public
  - *Secondary:* Triage, treatment, shelter supervision
  - *Tertiary:* Follow-up, recovery assistance, prevention of future disasters

Triage
The goal of triage is to maximize the number of survivors by sorting the injured as treatable and untreatable, using the criteria of potential for survival and availability of resources.
- Color-coded system
- START (simple *t*riage *a*nd *r*apid *t*reatment) method
- Identify the walking wounded; move them to an area where they can be evaluated later
- Three-step evaluation of others, done one at a time:
  - Respiration
  - Circulation
  - Mental status

The following clients present to the triage nurse in the emergency department (ED). Which client should the nurse ask the healthcare provider to see first?
A. A teary 19-year-old client with a temperature of 38.2° C (100.8° F) who has had vomiting and watery diarrhea five times in 3 hours.
B. A middle-aged client who has had a sore throat, swollen lymph nodes, and cough for 2 days and who had received the flu vaccine.
C. A 40-year-old client, brought to the ED by her co-workers, who has had a severe headache, vomiting, and a stiff neck for 48 hours. *risk of meningitis*
D. A 44-year-old client limping on a swollen ankle and complaining of ankle pain who has been self-medicating with Percocet (oxycodone/acetaminophen).

[Handwritten notes:]
Reopen airway…
If not breathing spontaneously, tag=black
If yes = Red
Resp. 730 = Red   ① normal = yellow
Cap refill dec. = Red   ② normal = yellow
Follow simple commands = yellow

HESI Test Question Approach		
Positive?	YES	NO
Key Words		
Rephrase		
Rule Out Choices		
A	B	C	D

Bioterrorism

Review exposure information, assessment findings, and treatment for various agents:

- Biological
- Chemical
- Radiation —*tracked longitudinally*

Exam questions may deal with disasters and bioterrorism as they affect the individual victim, families, and the community.

The nurse is completing discharge teaching for a group of postal employees who have been _exposed_ to a powder form of anthrax. Which instruction has the highest priority?

A. Begin the prescribed antibiotics and continue for 60 days.
B. Watch for symptoms of anthrax for the next 7 days.
C. Make arrangements to be vaccinated for anthrax.
D. Explain to family members that anthrax is not contagious.

Exposure to Anthrax= antibiotics 60 days

Sarin
Risin

HESI Test Question Approach		
Positive?	YES	NO
Key Words		
Rephrase		
Rule Out Choices		
A	B	C	D

5 Oxygenation, Ventilation, Transportation, and Perfusion

A client who is 1 day postoperative from a left pneumonectomy is lying on his right side with the head of the bed (HOB) elevated 10 degrees. The nurse assesses his respiratory rate at 32 breaths/min. What action should the nurse take first?

A. Further elevate the head of the bed
B. Assist the client into the supine position *(to allow functional lung to fully expand)*
C. Measure the client's O_2 saturation
D. Administer PRN morphine IV

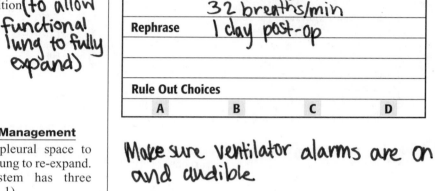

HESI Test Question Approach			
Positive?		YES	NO
Key Words	left		
	HOB 10 degrees		
	32 breaths/min		
Rephrase	1 day post-op		
Rule Out Choices			
A	B	C	D

Chest Tube and Water or Dry Seal Management

- Chest tubes are inserted into the pleural space to remove air and fluid and to allow the lung to re-expand.
- A chest collection drainage system has three compartments or chambers (Figure 5-1).
  — Collection chamber
    - Air and fluid are collected from the pleural or mediastinal space.
    - Fluid remains and air is vented to the second compartment, the water seal chamber.
  — Water seal chamber
    - This chamber contains 2 cm of water, which prevents backflow and acts as a one-way valve.
    - Fluctuations in the water level are known as *tidaling;* fluid should move upward with each inspiration and downward with each expiration.
  — Suction control chamber
    - Water suction uses 20 cm of water to aid in draining air or fluid from the chest.
    - Dry suction provides a safe and effective level of vacuum by continuously balancing the forces of suction and atmosphere.

Nursing and Collaborative Management

- Keep all tubing coiled loosely below chest level, with connections tight and taped.
- Monitor the fluid drainage and mark the time of measurement and the fluid level.
- Observe for air bubbling in the water seal chamber and fluctuations (tidaling).
- Replace the unit when full.
- Do not routinely clamp chest tubes.

Handwritten notes:

Make sure ventilator alarms are on and audible.

High-Volume Alarm
→ inc. spontaneous effort patient

Low-Volume Alarm
→ secretions in airway
  • suction patient
→ bronchospasm

Water in circuit (condensation)

Circuit disconnect

High Inspiratory Pressure
→ secretions
→ patient ventilator asynchrony "fighting the vent"; more sedation needed
→ circuit occlusion (pt. laying on tube, reposition)

Low Inspiratory Pressure
→ check for extubation
→ cuff leak (pt. can make sound)
→ circuit disconnect

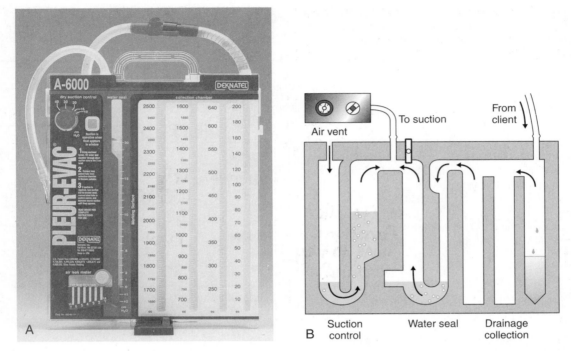

Figure 5-1 Chest drainage unit. Both units have three chambers: (1) collection chamber; (2) water-seal chamber; and (3) suction control chamber. Suction control chamber requires a connection to a wall suction source that is dialed to the prescribed suction A. Water suction. This unit uses water in the suction control chamber to control the wall suction pressure. B, Dry suction. This unit controls wall suction by using a regulator control dial. (From Lewis SL, et al: Medical-surgical nursing: Assessment and management of clinical problems, ed 7, St Louis, 2007, Mosby.)

- If the chest tube is accidentally dislodged, the nurse should:
  — Cover the area with a dry, sterile dressing
  — If an air leak is noted, tape the dressing on three sides only; this allows air to escape and prevents the formation of a tension pneumothorax
  — Notify the healthcare provider

Pneumonia

Pneumonia results in inflammation of lung tissue, causing consolidation of exudate.
- Pathogens
  — Bacterial (gram-negative is the most severe), viral, fungal (rare)
  — Community acquired or hospital acquired
- Host's physical status
- Aspiration
- Inhalation
- Hypostatic
- Anatomical areas
  — Lung parenchyma
  — Pleurae

Handwritten notes:

If chamber must be changed, put tube in cup of sterile water.
d/c
At⊗⊗, vaseline gauze and occlusive dressing.

(next to Aspiration) (elderly, infants, muscle weakness, dec. LOC) disorders

Aspiration precautions:
Thicken liquids
HOB elevated up to one hour
Mechanically soft diet
check residuals
open airway

The spouse of a 94-year-old client reports to the home health nurse that his wife has become increasingly confused over the past few days and has developed a cough. Which assessment should the nurse perform first?

A. Jugular vein distention
B. Skin turgor
C. Oxygen saturation — *confusion, and lack of oxygen is often the first sign of pneumonia*
D. Pupillary response to light

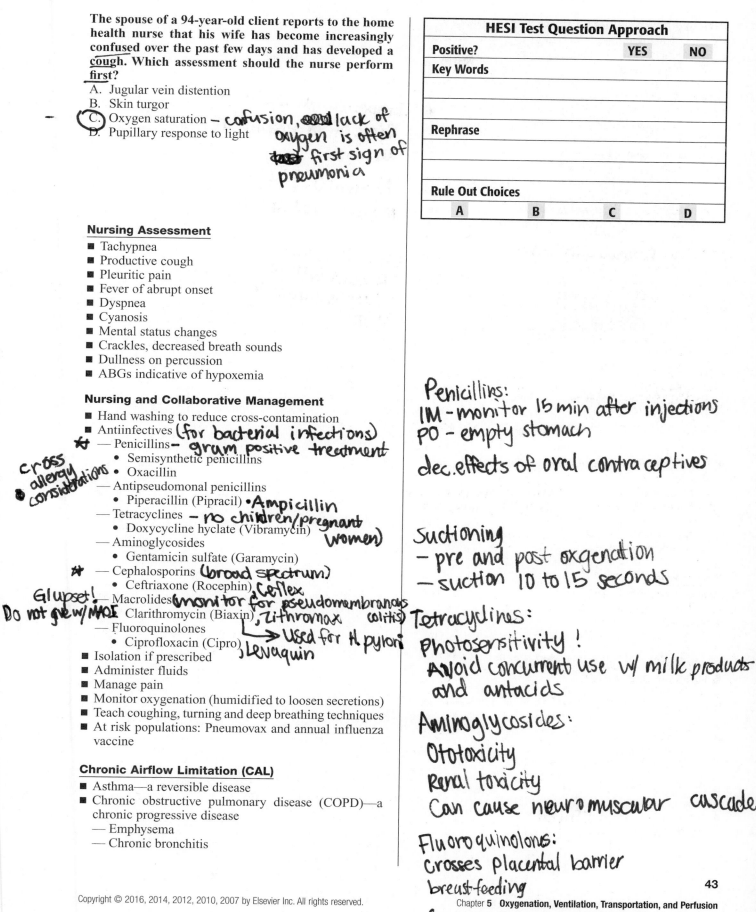

HESI Test Question Approach

Positive?		YES	NO
Key Words			
Rephrase			
Rule Out Choices			
A	B	C	D

Nursing Assessment

- Tachypnea
- Productive cough
- Pleuritic pain
- Fever of abrupt onset
- Dyspnea
- Cyanosis
- Mental status changes
- Crackles, decreased breath sounds
- Dullness on percussion
- ABGs indicative of hypoxemia

Nursing and Collaborative Management

- Hand washing to reduce cross-contamination
- Antiinfectives *(for bacterial infections)*
  - Penicillins— *gram positive treatment*
    - Semisynthetic penicillins
    - Oxacillin
  - Antipseudomonal penicillins
    - Piperacillin (Pipracil) • *Ampicillin*
  - Tetracyclines — *no children/pregnant women*
    - Doxycycline hyclate (Vibramycin)
  - Aminoglycosides
    - Gentamicin sulfate (Garamycin)
  - Cephalosporins *(broad spectrum)*
    - Ceftriaxone (Rocephin) *Ceflex*
  - Macrolides *monitor for pseudomembranous colitis*
    - Clarithromycin (Biaxin), *Zithromax*
  - Fluoroquinolones
    - Ciprofloxacin (Cipro) *) Levaquin* → *Used for H. pylori*
- Isolation if prescribed
- Administer fluids
- Manage pain
- Monitor oxygenation (humidified to loosen secretions)
- Teach coughing, turning and deep breathing techniques
- At risk populations: Pneumovax and annual influenza vaccine

cross allergy considerations
GI upset!
Do not give w/ MAOI

Chronic Airflow Limitation (CAL)

- Asthma—a reversible disease
- Chronic obstructive pulmonary disease (COPD)—a chronic progressive disease
  - Emphysema
  - Chronic bronchitis

Penicillins:
IM - monitor 15 min after injections
PO - empty stomach
dec. effects of oral contraceptives

Suctioning
- pre and post oxgenation
- suction 10 to 15 seconds

Tetracyclines:
Photosensitivity!
Avoid concurrent use w/ milk products and antacids

Aminoglycosides:
Ototoxicity
Renal toxicity
Can cause neuromuscular cascade

Fluoroquinolones:
Crosses placental barrier
breast-feeding
Can lower seizure threshold

Etiology and Precipitating Factors for COPD

- Cigarette smoking
- Environmental/occupational exposure
- Genetic predisposition

Chronic Bronchitis

- Pathophysiology
  — Chronic sputum with cough production on a daily basis for a minimum of 3 months/year
  — Chronic hypoxemia/cor pulmonale
  — Increased mucus, cilia production
  — Increased bronchial wall thickness (obstructs air flow)
  — Exacerbations usually due to infection
  — Increased CO_2 retention/acidemia
  — Reduced responsiveness of respiratory center to hypoxemic stimuli

— Inc. pressure in lung

Emphysema

- Abnormal enlargement of the air spaces distal to the terminal alveolar walls
- Increased dyspnea/work of breathing
  — Reduced gas exchange surface area
  — Increased air trapping (increased anterior-posterior diameter)
  — Decreased capillary network
  — Increased work/increased O_2 consumption

— Work to reduce

Nursing Assessment: COPD

- Inspection
  — Bronchitis
    • Right-sided heart failure
    • Cyanosis distended neck veins
  — Emphysema
    • Pursed-lip breathing
    • Noncyanotic, thin   *• diminished breath sounds; wheezes*
- Auscultation
  — Bronchitis
    • Crackles
    • Rhonchi
    • Expiratory wheezes
  — Emphysema
    • Distant breath sounds
    • Quiet breath sounds
    • Wheezes

Nursing and Collaborative Management: COPD

- Lowest O_2 to prevent CO_2 retention
  — Take particular care not to abolish the hypoxic drive needed for effective breathing if the client has COPD and is known to retain CO_2.
  — Obtain parameters for acceptable O_2 saturation levels.
- Monitor for signs and symptoms (S/S) of fluid overload.
- Baseline ABGs for CO_2 retainers.
- Teach the client pursed-lip breathing.
- Orthopneic position *(Tripod)*

— opens up chest wall

Handwritten notes (right margin):

Impaired gas exchange
Risk of respiratory acidosis

Normal O_2 sat. could be around 90

Cor Pulmonale
- R. heart failure
- liver enlargement
- JVD

An elderly man comes to the emergency department (ED) complaining of shortness of breath. The healthcare provider (HCP) determines that the client has pneumonia. The client's condition deteriorates in the ED, and he now has impending respiratory failure. Which set of arterial blood gas (ABG) values demonstrates acute respiratory failure?

A) pH–7.30 Pco_2–52 • Po_2–56 Hco_3–26
B. pH–7.35 Pco_2–44 Po_2–86 Hco_3–28
C. pH–7.35 Pco_2–62 Po_2–66 Hco_3–31
D. pH–7.30 Pco_2–39 Po_2–88 Hco_3–22

[handwritten: PO_2 <60 indicates resp. failure. check for compensation]

Reactive Airway Disease
Asthma

Asthma is an inflammatory disorder of the airways characterized by an exaggerated bronchoconstrictor response to a wide variety of stimuli.

- Allergens
- Environmental irritants
- Cold air
- Exercise
- β-blockers
- Respiratory infection
- Emotional stress
- Reflux esophagitis

Drug Therapy for Asthma and COPD
Bronchodilators

- Long-acting inhaled $β_2$-adrenergic agonists
- Long-acting oral $β_2$-adrenergic agonists
- Theophylline (Theolair, Uniphyl)
- Short-acting inhaled $β_2$-adrenergic agonists
- Anticholinergics (inhaled)

$β_2$-Adrenergic Agonists

- Inhaled: Short Acting
  — Metaproterenol (Alupent, Metaprel): nebulizer, oral tablets, elixir, metered-dose inhaler (MDI)
  — Salbutamol sulfate (Albuterol, Proventil, Apo-Salvent, Ventolin HFA, Volmax): nebulizer, MDI, oral tablets, Rotahaler
  — Levalbuterol (Xopenex, Xopenex HFA): nebulizer, MDI
  — Terbutaline (Bricanyl, Brethine): oral tablets, nebulizer, subcutaneous, MDI
  — Bitolterol (Tornalate): MDI, nebulizer
- Inhaled: Long Acting
  — Salmeterol xinofoate (Serevent): dry powder inhaler (DPI)
  — Formoterol fumurate (Foradil): DPI
- Immediate Acting
  — Epinephrine hydrochloride (Adrenalin chloride): subcutaneous

HESI Test Question Approach

Positive?		YES	NO
Key Words	*acute respiratory failure*		
Rephrase			
Rule Out Choices			
A	B	C	D

[handwritten: Body inc. cardiac output when faced w/ stressors.]

- Corticosteroids
  - Hydrocortisone (Solu-Cortef): IV
  - Methylprednisolone (Solu-Medrol): IV
  - Prednisone: oral
  - Beclomethasone dipropionate (Gen-Beclo AQ, Vanceril, Beclovent, Vanceril DS, Qvar, Qvar HFA): inhaler
  - Triamcinolone acetonide (Nasacort AQ Azmacort): inhaler
  - Fluticasone furoate (Avamys): inhaler
  - Fluticasone propionate (Flonase, Flovent HFA, Flovent Diskus): inhaler
  - Budesonide (Pulmicort Turbuhaler, Pulmicort Nebuamp, Rhinocort Aqua, Rhinocort Turbuhaler): inhaler
  - Mometasone furoate monohydrate (Nasonex): inhaler
- Anticholinergics
  - Short-acting ipratropium bromide (Atrovent): nebulizer, MDI
  - Long-acting tiotropium (Spiriva): DPI
- Mast Cell Stabilizers (rarely used)
  - Cromolyn sodium
  - Nedocromil sodium
- IgE Antagonist
  - Omalizumab (Xolair): subcutaneous injection
- Leukotriene Modifiers
  - Leukotriene receptor blockers
    - Zafirlukast (Accolate): oral tablets
    - Montelukast sodium (Singulair): oral tablets, chewable tablets, oral granules
  - Leukotriene inhibitor
    - Zileuton (Zyflo): oral tablets
- Methylxanthines
  - Aminophylline as an IV agent is rarely used. Available as oral, rectal, injectable, and topical.
  - Oral: Elixophyllin, Quibron, Slo-bid, Theochron, Theolair, Theo-24, Uniphyl
- Combination Agents
  - Ipratropium and salbutamol (Combivent): MDI, nebulizer
  - Fluticasone propionate/salmeterol (Advair Diskus): DPI

Nursing Assessment
- Dyspnea, wheezing, chest tightness
- Assess precipitating factors
- Medication history

Nursing and Collaborative Management
- Monitor respirations and assess breath sounds
- Monitor oxygen saturation
- Monitor mental status
- Chest physiotherapy
- Assess peripheral pulses and warmth and color of extremities
- Position for maximum ventilation
- Encourage slow, pursed-lip breathing
- Encourage abdominal breathing
- Administer humidified oxygen therapy

Handwritten margin notes:
- Rinse mouth after treatment to prevent candidiasis
- Relaxation of bronchial muscles
- Taken to prevent asthma attack
- Use of a spacer
- Try to discover trigger

46

The nurse palpates a crackling sensation of the skin around the insertion site of a chest tube in a client who has had thoracic surgery. What action should the nurse take?

A. Return the client to surgery
B. Prepare for insertion of a larger chest tube
C. Increase the water seal suction pressure
D. Continue to monitor the insertion site

Small amount of crepitus expected; mark extent and monitor

HESI Test Question Approach		
Positive?	**YES**	**NO**
Key Words		
Rephrase		
Rule Out Choices		
A	B	C	D

Pulmonary Tuberculosis (TB)

TB is a communicable lung disease caused by the bacillus *Mycobacterium tuberculosis* or the tubercle bacillus, an acid-fast organism that is spread by airborne transmission.

Resurgence of TB
- Related to HIV infection
- Multidrug-resistant TB (MDR-TB)
  — Rifampin
  — Isoniazid
- Seen disproportionately in poor, underserved, and minorities

Nursing Assessment
- Low-grade fever
- Pallor
- Chills
- Night sweats
- Easy fatigability
- Anorexia
- Weight loss

Should be reported.

Nursing and Collaborative Management
- Airborne precautions isolation
  — Single-occupancy room with negative pressure and airflow of 6 to 12 exchanges per hour
- Wear high-efficiency particulate air (HEPA) masks
- Teach client to cover the nose and mouth with paper tissues whenever coughing, sneezing, or producing sputum.
- Emphasize careful hand washing after handling sputum and soiled tissues.
- If client needs to be out of the negative-pressure room, he or she must wear a standard isolation mask to prevent exposure to others.
- Medication regimen
  — Isoniazid (INH therapy)
  — Pyridoxine (vitamin B6)
  — Rifampin (Rifadin, Rofact)
  — Pyrazinamide
  — With or without streptomycin and ethambutol (Etibi)
  — Take as prescribed for 9 to 12 months
  — Teach client the side effects

Acid Fast Bacillus Test (AFB)
→ *neg. 4 days is goal*

sweat, tears orange

TB Drugs and Side Effects
First-Line Drugs
First-line drugs are bacteriocidal against rapidly dividing cells and/or against semidormant bacteria.

- Isoniazid (INH): clinical hepatitis, fulminant hepatitis, peripheral neurotoxicity
- Rifampin (Rifadin, Rofact): cutaneous reactions, GI disturbance (nausea, anorexia, abdominal pain), flulike syndrome, hepatotoxicity, immunological reactions, orange discoloration of bodily fluids (sputum, urine, sweat, tears)
- Ethambutol hydrochloride (Myambutol, Etibi): retrobulbar neuritis (decreased red-green color discrimination), skin rash
- Rifabutin (Mycobutin): hematologic toxicity, GI symptoms, polyarthralgias, pseudojaundice, orange discoloration of bodily fluids
- Pyrazinamide (PZA): hepatotoxicity, GI symptoms (nausea, vomiting), polyarthralgias, skin rash, hyperuricemia, dermatitis

Second-Line Drugs
Second-line drugs are bactericidal and/or bacteriostatic and/or inhibits cell wall synthesis.

- Cycloserine (Seromycin): CNS effects; given with pyridoxine to prevent neurotoxic effects
- Ethionamide (Trecator): hepatotoxicity, neurotoxicity, GI effects (metallic taste, nausea, vomiting), endocrine effects (hypothyroidism, impotence)
- Streptomycin sulfate: ototoxicity, neurotoxicity, nephrotoxicity
- Amikacin sulfate and kanamycin: ototoxicity, nephrotoxicity
- Para-aminosalicylic acid (PAS): hepatotoxicity, GI distress, malabsorption syndrome, coagulopathy
- Fluoroquinolones (levofloxacin [Levaquin, moxifloxacin hydrochloride [Avelox, Vigamox], gatifloxacin [Tequin]): GI disturbances, neurological effects (dizziness, headaches) rash

Pulmonary Embolus
Any substance can cause an embolism. Typically, a blood clot enters the venous circulation and lodges in the pulmonary vasculature.

Risk Factors for VTE Leading to PE
- Prolonged immobility
- Central venous catheters
- Surgery
- Obesity
- Advancing age
- Conditions that increase blood clotting
- History of thromboembolism
- Smoking, BCP, pregnancy

Signs and Symptoms
- Dyspnea
- Sharp, stabbing chest pain
- Apprehension, restlessness

Monitor for compliance

48

- Feeling of impending doom ✿
- Cough
- Hemoptysis
- Tachypnea
- Crackles
- Pleural friction rub
- Tachycardia
- S3 or S4 heart sound
- Diaphoresis
- Low-grade fever
- Decreased arterial oxygen saturation (Sao_2); respiratory alkalosis, then respiratory acidosis
- Diagnosed by findings, and computed tomography (CT) scans, transesophageal echocardiography (TEE)

Nursing and Collaborative Management
Prevention
- Range-of-motion exercises
- Ambulate and turn
- Use antiembolism and pneumatic compression stockings
- Assess peripheral circulation
- Administer prescribed prophylactic low-dose anticoagulant and antiplatelet drugs
- Teach client and family about precautions
  — Encourage client to stop smoking

Acute Management
- Oxygen therapy
- Monitor ABG studies and pulse oximetry
- Check vital signs, lung sounds, and cardiac and respiratory status
- Anticoagulants are used to prevent embolus enlargement and the formation of new clots; use with caution with active bleeding, stroke, and recent trauma
  — Heparin is usually used unless the PE is massive or occurs with hemodynamic instability
  — Alteplase (Activase, tPA, Cathflo), fibrinolytic drugs
    • Therapeutic PTT values usually range from 1.5 to 2.5 times
    • Both heparin and fibrinolytic drugs are high-alert drugs
- Embolectomy
- Inferior vena cava filtration with placement of a vena cava filter

Hematological Problems
Anemia
- Etiology
  — Decreased erythrocyte production
  — Decreased hemoglobin synthesis
    • Iron deficiency anemia
- Defective DNA synthesis
  — Vitamin B_{12} deficiency
  — Folic acid deficiency
- Decreased number of erythrocyte precursors
  — Aplastic anemia

Oral contraceptives raise risk of developing blood clot

Ticlit, Plavix anti-platelets

- Chronic diseases or disorders
- Chemotherapy
- Blood loss
  — Acute
  — Trauma
- Blood vessel rupture
- Chronic gastritis
- Menstrual flow
- Hemorrhoids

Nursing Assessment

- Pallor
- Fatigue
- Exercise intolerance
- Tachycardia *(body trying to compensate)*
- Dyspnea
- Assess for risk factors
  — Diet low in iron, vitamin B_{12} deficiency, history of bleeding, medications taken
  — Hgb <100 mmol/L (10 g/dL), Hct <0.36 volume fraction (36%), RBCs $<4 \times 10^{12}$/L

Nursing Interventions

- Treatment of underlying pathology
- Administer blood products as prescribed
- Encourage diet high in iron-rich foods, folic acid, vitamin B_{12}, vitamin B_6, amino acids, and vitamin C
- Give parenteral iron via **Z**-track technique

or oral supplements

Blood Transfusions
Blood Groups and Types

- ABO system includes A, B, O, and AB blood types.
- Rh factor is an antigenic substance in the erythrocytes.
- If blood is mismatched during transfusion, a transfusion reaction occurs.
  — Transfusion reaction is an antigen-antibody reaction.
  — It can range from a mild response to severe anaphylactic shock.

Types of Reactions

- Acute hemolytic
- Febrile, nonhemolytic (most common)
- Mild allergic
- Anaphylactic
- Delayed hemolytic

Types of Blood Products

- Red blood cells (RBCs)
  - Packed RBCs (PRBCs)
  - Autologous PRBCs
  - Washed RBCs
  - Frozen RBCs
  - Leukocyte-poor RBCs
  - RBC units with high number of reticulocytes (young RBCs)
- Other cellular components
  - Platelets
  - Granulocytes
- Plasma components
  - Fresh frozen plasma (FFP)
  - Cryoprecipitate
  - Serum albumin
  - Plasma protein fraction (PPF)
  - Immune serum globulin

Nursing Interventions

- Perform assessment before, during, and after transfusion, including the IV site
- Two identifiers
- Confirm informed consent
- Identify the compatibility
- Initiate a transfusion slowly, then maintain the infusion rate
  - 1 unit of PRBCs is transfused in 2 to 4 hours

A client who is receiving a transfusion of packed red blood cells has an inflamed IV site. What action should the nurse take?

A. Double-check with another nurse the blood type of the transfusing unit of blood

B. Discontinue the transfusion and send the remaining blood and tubing to the lab

C. Immediately start a new IV at another site and resume the transfusion at the new site

D. Continue to monitor the site for signs of infection and notify the healthcare provider

Inflamed IV site does not indicate ~~allergic rx~~ transfusion

Hypertension (HTN)

- Persistent BP elevation > 140/90 mmHg
- Risk factors
  - Nonmodifiable: family history, gender, age, ethnicity
  - Modifiable: use of alcohol, tobacco, caffeine; sedentary lifestyle; obesity

If rx occurs, stop the infusion and flush IV site w/ NS
- detach tubing w/ blood

HESI Test Question Approach			
Positive?		**YES**	**NO**
Key Words			
Rephrase			
Rule Out Choices			
A	**B**	**C**	**D**

Medications

- Diuretics → reduces volume in vasculature
  — Thiazides, Metolazone Zaroxolyn
- Antihypertensives
  — Prazosin hydrochloride Minipress, Atenolol (Tenormin), Clonidine (Catapres)
- ACE inhibitors → vasodilate, lowers BP (cough)
  — Lisinopril (Zestril), captopril
- Calcium channel blockers → block Ca⁺ influx
  — Diltiazem hydrochloride (Cardizem)
  - slows conduction thru AV node; dilate arteries

HTN Education

- The number one cause of stroke (cerebrovascular accident, CVA) is nonadherence to HTN medications.

- diet, exercise, smoking cessation, alcohol modification

Clonidine relaxes smooth muscle in body; reduces BP
- rebound htn
- for emergent situations

Beta-Blockers:
- olol (metoprolol...)
- block stress response
- dec. HR & contractility
- blocks bronchodilation
- negative inotrope

ARBs:
- Losartan
- If pt. cannot take ACE

ACE inhibitors prevent ventricular remodeling

Coronary Artery Disease (CAD)

- Prevalent etiologies of CAD
  — Atherosclerosis: Partially or completely blocked coronary arteries
  — Coronary vasospasm (Heroin & cocaine abusers)
  — Microvascular angina
- CAD results in ischemia and infarction of myocardial tissue.
- Left anterior descending artery (LAD) is most commonly affected.
  CAD "Widow maker"

CAD is one of the leading causes of morbidity and mortality among adults in Canada and remains the number one health problem in the United States.

Reduction of Risk Factors

- Stop smoking
- Lose weight
- Decrease blood pressure
- Increase activity/exercise

Angina

- Varies from mild to severe, transient to prolonged
- Gradual or sudden onset
- May radiate to either arm and to shoulder, jaw, neck, or epigastric area
- *Other S/S*: dyspnea, tachycardia, palpitations, nausea and vomiting, fatigue, diaphoresis, pallor, syncope, SOB (esp. in elderly)
- Usually subsides with rest or nitroglycerin
- Often precipitated by exercise, cold exposure, heavy meal, stress, intercourse

Vasodilators can cause headaches.

Nitrates + Viagra can lead to stage 3 shock (within 48hrs)

Diet Therapy
- Dietary modification
- Goal is to reduce serum cholesterol and serum triglycerides
- Maintain ideal body weight
- Daily cholesterol intake should be restricted to <200 mg/day

Drug Classes for Angina Management
- **Antiplatelet agents**
  — Acetylsalicylic acid (ASA, aspirin)
  — Clopidogrel (Plavix)
- **β-blockers**
  — Atenolol (Tenormin)
  — Metoprolol tartrate (Lopressor, Betaloc)
- **Nitrates**
  — Nitroglycerin
  — Isosorbide dinitrate
  — Sodium Nitroprusside
- **Calcium channel blockers**
  — Diltiazem (Cardizem)
  — Verapamil hydrochloride
- **Thrombolytics**
  — Alteplase (recombinant t-PA) (Activase, Cathflo)
  — Reteplase (Retavase)
  — Tenecteplase (TNKase)
  — Streptokinase (SK, Streptase)
- **Anticoagulants**
  — Unfractionated heparin
  — Low-molecular-weight heparin (LMWH) (enoxaparin sodium [Lovenox])
- **ACE inhibitors**
  — Captopril (Capoten)
  — Enalapril sodium (Vasotec)
  — Benazepril hydrochloride (Lotensin)
- **Analgesics**
  — Morphine sulfate

Cholesterol-Lowering Drugs
These drugs may be initiated if dietary modification is unsuccessful.
- Atorvastatin calcium (Lipitor)
- Lovastatin (Mevacor)
- Pravastatin sodium (Pravasa, Pravachol)
- Rosuvastatin calcium (Crestor)
- Simvastatin (Zocor)
- Ezetimibe (Ezetrol)
- Gemfibrozil (Lopid)
- Nicotinic acid (Niacin)

Oxygen
- Administer at 4 to 6 L/min to assist in oxygenating myocardial tissue

→ Cholesterol reduction:
diet/exercise
Statins
Niacin (aspirin minimizes flushing of face)

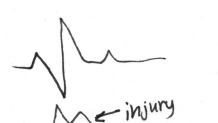

← injury (ST elevation)

← ischemia (T-wave inversion)

← necrosis (pathologic Q) Not everyone presents w/ acute infarction

90 min. window to prevent LV damage

Angioplasty & stent preferred to thrombolytic

Nitroglycerin

- Dilates the coronary arteries
- Increases blood flow to the damaged area of myocardium
- Dosage
  — 0.4 mg/tablet
  — 1 tab sublingual q 5 min × 3 doses

Morphine Sulfate

- Analgesic
- ↓ Anxiety and tachypnea
- Relaxes bronchial smooth muscle
- Improves gas exchange

Thrombolytic Therapy

- Useful when infarction is diagnosed early and administered within protocol guidelines. There is a time imperative.
- Streptokinase or Alteplase or tPA
  — Administered IV
  — Most effective if given within 6 hours of onset of chest pain
- Heparin therapy usually follows thrombolytic therapy.

β-Blockers

- Decrease heart rate
- Reduce workload of the heart
- Decrease oxygen demand of myocardium

Calcium Channel Blockers

- Decrease conduction through AV node
- Slow heart rate
- Decrease oxygen demand by myocardium

Medical Interventions

- Percutaneous transluminal coronary angioplasty (PTCA)
  — Balloon angioplasty
- Intracoronary stents
- Coronary artery bypass graft (CABG)

Acute Myocardial Infarction

- Destruction of myocardial tissue due to lack of blood and oxygen supply
- Begins with occlusion of the coronary artery
- Ischemia, injury, infarction

Ischemia

- Results from reduced blood flow and oxygen to the coronary arteries
- If not reversed, injury occurs
- Ischemia lasting 20 minutes or longer is sufficient to produce irreversible tissue damage.

Injury

- Prolonged interruption of oxygen supply and nutrients
- Cells still salvageable

Aspirin given

Infarction

- Tissue necrosis and death
- Irreversible damage
- Scar tissue has no electrical stimulation or contractility.
- Within 24 hours of infarction, healing process begins.

Complications

- As many as 90% of clients suffer complications, including:
  — Dysrhythmias
  — Cardiac failure
  — Cardiogenic shock
  — Thromboembolism
  — Ventricular rupture

Signs and Symptoms

- Pain
  — Sudden onset; severity increases
  — May persist for hours or days; not relieved by rest or nitroglycerin
  — Heavy/constrictive
  — Located behind the sternum
  — May radiate to arms, back, neck, or jaw
- Cool, clammy skin
- Rapid, irregular, feeble pulse

Atypical Symptoms

- Women
  — Discomfort rather than pain
  — Shortness of breath
  — Extreme fatigue
- Client with diabetes
  — May be asymptomatic
  — Neuropathy
  — Dyspnea
- Elderly client
  — Confusion/delirium
  — Dizziness
  — Shortness of breath

Medical Diagnosis

- ECG (12 lead) – ST segment elevation, T-wave inversion, pathologic Q-wave formation
- Confirm by cardiac biomarkers
  — CK-MB
  — Myoglobin
  — Troponin

Cardiac Lab Tests

- Troponin level
  — Troponins are found only in cardiac muscle.
  — May present as early after injury
  — Peaks within 24 hours
  — Returns to normal in 5 to 14 days
- Myoglobin level *normally <90*
  — Myoglobin is released 1 hour after an acute myocardial infarction (MI).
  — Rises before creatine kinase–MB levels
  — Returns to normal within 24 hours

CkMB >5
Trop I > 0.1
Trop II > 0.1 } *indicative of Myocardial damage*
Myoglobin > 90

Treatment

- Overall goal is to preserve myocardial tissue.
- Drug therapy
  — Oxygen
  — Nitroglycerin
  — Morphine
  — Thrombolytic therapy
  — Other medications
- Angioplasty and stents
  — Used when drug therapy is not successful
- Coronary artery bypass graft
  — Used for severe coronary artery disease
  — Can be emergent or elective procedure

Heart Failure

Etiology

- CAD, prior MI
- Chronic HTN
- Cardiomyopathy
  — Dilated
- Idiopathic
- Thyroid
- Diabetes
  — Restrictive
  — Ischemic
- Valvular and congenital heart disease
- Pulmonary diseases

Left-Sided Heart Failure (LHF)

- *Causes:* LV infarct, cardiomyopathy
- *Symptoms:* dyspnea, cough, fluid accumulation in the lungs
- *Signs:* S3 gallop, tachycardia, inspiratory rales beginning at lung bases, expiratory wheezes due to bronchospasms (misdiagnosed with asthma)
- *Laboratory findings:* ABGs reveal hypoxemia; chest radiograph shows pulmonary edema or pleural effusions

Right-Sided Heart Failure (RHF) Systemic Congestion

- *Causes:* LHF, RV infarct, pulmonary or tricuspid valve disease, pulmonary HTN, COPD, PE
- *Symptoms:* dyspnea on exertion, fatigue, weight gain, fluid retention
- *Signs:* increased central venous pressure (CVP), jugular venous distention (JVD) > 3 to 4 cm, hepatomegaly, ascites, peripheral or sacral edema; pleural and pericardial effusions are also not uncommon

Sodium and Volume Homeostasis

- As CO decreases, renal perfusion decreases.
- This activates the renin-angiotensin system.
- This causes fluid retention.

RHF Laboratory Tests

- Liver function shows hepatic congestion
- Increased liver enzymes, increased PT, INR
- Hyponatremia (fluid restriction only if Na^+ < 132 mmol/L (mEq/L)
- Increased BUN/creatinine = decreased renal perfusion

S3 Ken-tuck-y
S4 — Tenn-e-see

56

Pharmacological Management

- **Angiotensin-converting enzyme (ACE) inhibitors** *(Vasodilate)*
  - Captopril
  - Enalapril sodium
  - Fosinopril sodium
  - Lisinopril
  - Quinapril hydrochloride
  - Ramipril
  - Perindopril erbumine
  - Benazepril hydrochloride
- **Diuretics**
  - Loop diuretics
    - Furosemide
    - Bumetanide
- **Thiazides**
  - Thiazide-related drug: metolazone
- **Aldosterone antagonists**
  - Spironolactone
- **Inotropes** *(inc. contractility)*
  - Digoxin
  - Dobutamine hydrochloride
- **Phosphodiesterase inhibitors**
  - Milrinone
- **Natriuretic peptides**
  - Nesiritide
- **β-blockers** *(dec. workload on ♥)*
  - Metoprolol
  - Carvedilol
  - Bisoprolol
- **Angiotensin II receptor blockers** *(if pt. cannot tolerate ACE)*
  - Losartan potassium
  - Candesartan cilexetil
  - Valsartan
- **Vasodilators**
  - Nitrates: isosorbide dinitrate
  - Hydralazine hydrochloride
  - Sodium nitroprusside
  - Prazosin hydrochloride
- **Dopamine agonist**
  - Dopamine hydrochloride
- **Analgesics**
  - Morphine sulfate
- **Anticoagulants**
  - Warfarin
- **Antiplatelet**
  - Aspirin

Nursing and Collaborative Management

- Activity
  - Regular exercise strongly encouraged—improves function of skeletal muscle more than changes in myocardial function
- Diet
  - Limit sodium intake
  - Fluid restriction only if $Na^+ < 132$ mmol/L (mEq/L)
  - Avoid excessive fluids
  - Avoid alcohol—depresses myocardial contractility
  - With CAD: low cholesterol, low fat, low Na^+

The nurse is administering 0900 medications to three clients on a telemetry unit when the UAP reports that another client is complaining of a sudden onset of substernal discomfort. What action should the nurse take?

A. Ask the UAP to obtain the client's VS
B. Assess the client's discomfort *(could potentially be MI)*
C. Advise the client to rest in bed
D. Observe the client's ECG pattern

PEA possible
infarction may happen in different lead
Patient first!

HESI Test Question Approach		
Positive?	YES	NO
Key Words		
Rephrase		
Rule Out Choices		
A	B	C	D

A 62-year-old client who has a history of coronary heart disease was admitted to the acute care unit 2 days ago for management of angina. During the assessment, the client states, "I feel like I have indigestion." In what order should the nurse implement care? (Arrange from first action to last.)

4 A. Notify the rapid response team
3 B. Administer PRN nitroglycerin prescription
1 C. Check the pulse, respirations, blood pressure, and oxygen saturation *(baseline vitals)*
5 D. Document assessment on the electronic medical record
2 E. Provide 2 L of oxygen via nasal cannula

HESI Test Question Approach		
Positive?	YES	NO
Key Words		
Rephrase		
Rule Out Choices		
A	B	C	D

A client complains of a severe headache after receiving nitroglycerin 0.4 mg SL for angina. What prescription should the nurse administer?

A. A second dose of nitroglycerin
B. A scheduled dose of low-dose aspirin
C. A PRN dose of acetaminophen PO
D. A PRN dose of morphine sulfate IV

HESI Test Question Approach		
Positive?	YES	NO
Key Words		
Rephrase		
Rule Out Choices		
A	B	C	D

Dysrhythmias: Interpretation and Management
- Standard ECG (12 leads)
  — Provides best overall evaluation
- Telemetry
  — Usually three leads show one view of the heart
- Holter monitor
  — Usually, worn by client to obtain a 24-hour continuous reading

Event
—1-2 mo period of time
—press button when chest pain is felt

Electrocardiogram (ECG)

- P wave
  - — Atrial depolarization
- QRS complex
  - — Ventricular depolarization
  - — Normal: <0.11 second
- ST segment
  - — Early ventricular repolarization
- P-R interval
  - — Reflects time required for impulse to travel through SA node
  - — Normal: 0.12 to 0.20 second
- R-R interval
  - — Reflects regularity of heartbeat

Dysrhythmias

- Client may be asymptomatic until cardiac output is altered.
- Client may complain of palpitations, syncope, pain, dyspnea, diaphoresis.
- Changes seen in pulse rate/rhythm, as well as ECG changes.
- Always treat the client, *not* the monitor.

Atrial Dysrhythmias

- A-fib (atrial fibrillation)
  - — Chaotic activity in the AV node
  - — No true P waves visible
  - — Irregular ventricular rhythm
  - — Risk for CVA
  - — Anticoagulant therapy required
- Atrial flutter
  - — Sawtoothed waveform
  - — Fluttering in the chest
  - — Ventricular rhythm regular
- Cardioversion may be used to treat either type of atrial dysrhythmia.

Ventricular Dysrhythmias

- V-tach (ventricular tachycardia)
  - — Wide, bizarre QRS complex
  - — Assess whether client has a pulse
  - — Is cardiac output impaired?
  - — Prepare for synchronized cardioversion
  - — Administer antiarrhythmic drugs
- V-fib (ventricular fibrillation)
  - — Cardiac emergency
  - — No cardiac output
  - — Start cardiopulmonary resuscitation (CPR)
  - — Defibrillate as quickly as possible
  - — Administer antiarrhythmic drugs

Antiarrhythmic Medications

- **Class I:** sodium channel blockers (decrease conduction velocity in the atria, ventricles, and His-Purkinje system)
  - — **IA**
    - Disopyramide
    - Procainamide hydrochloride (Procan SR)
    - Quinidine sulfate

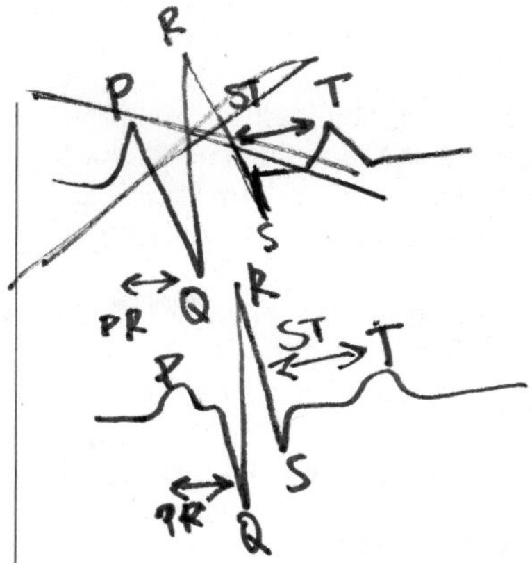

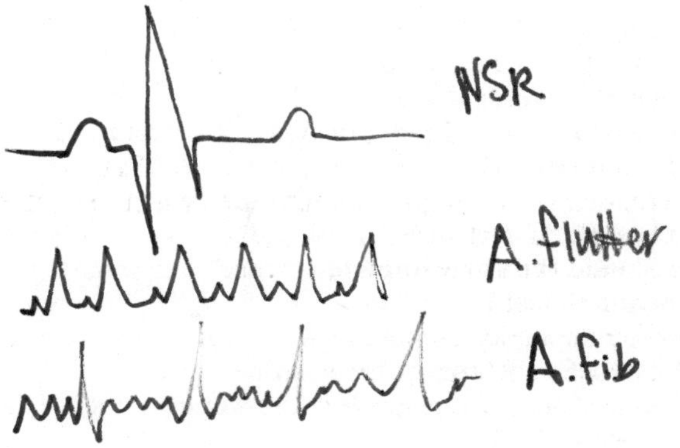

Handwritten annotations:

R P ST T S PR Q R ST T P S PR Q

NSR

A. flutter

A. fib

Atrial kick is lost.
CO dec. (30%)
No synchronous contraction.

① Check for pulse and stability of rhythm
② Systolic BP (100)
③ LOC to check for brain perfusion
Skin, chest pain, breathing rhythm
⑥ ④ ⑤ SOB

defib. as quickly as possible (pulseless)

defibrillate

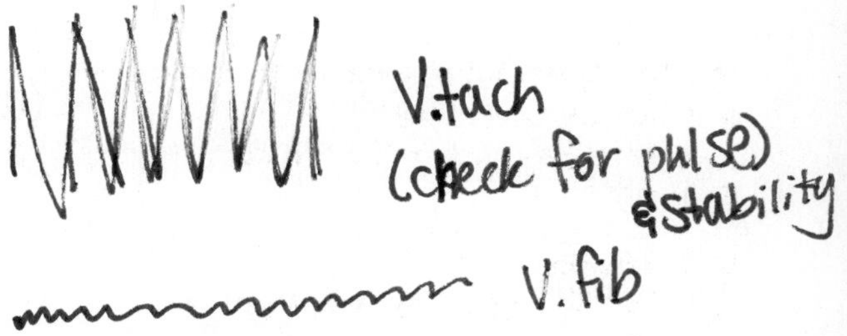

V. tach (check for pulse) & stability

V. fib

59

— **IB**
  - Lidocaine hydrochloride (Xylocaine)
  - Mexiletine hydrochloride
  - Phenytoin sodium (Dilantin)
— **IC**
  - Flecainide acetate (Tambocor)
  - Propafenone hydrochloride (Rythmol)
— **Other Class I**
  - Moricizine
- **Class II:** β-adrenergic blockers (decrease automaticity of the SA node, decrease conduction velocity in AV node)
  — Acebutolol hydrochloride (Rhotrol, Sectral)
  — Atenolol (Tenormin)
  — Esmolol hydrochloride (Brevibloc)
  — Metoprolol tartrate (Lopressor)
  — Sotalol hydrochloride (Rylosol)
- **Class III:** potassium channel blockers (delay repolarization)
  — Amiodarone hydrochloride (supported by EBP for atrial & ventricular)
  — Dofetilide (Tikosyn)
  — Sotalol hydrochloride (Betapace)
- **Class IV:** calcium channel blockers (decrease automaticity of SA node, delay AV node conduction)
  — Diltiazem hydrochloride (Cardizem)
  — Verapamil hydrochloride (Apo-Verap, Covera-HS, Isoptin SR

add cardizem to control HR

Handwritten margin notes:
QT <0.44 sec
Anti-arhythmics prolonge refractory period
SVT
— adenosine (cardioverter; 2 sec half life)
— cough/bear down (vagel)
[stops the heart for a second]

Other Antidysrhythmic Drugs
- Adenosine (Adenocard)
- Digoxin (Lanoxin)
- Ibutilide fumarate (Corvert)
- Magnesium

A 60-year-old client who has a history of hypertension, heart failure, and sleep apnea is admitted to the acute care unit. Which finding(s) would relate most directly to a diagnosis of acute decompensated heart failure? (Select all that apply.)
A. Respiratory rate of 25 breaths/min
B. Orthopnea
C. S3 heart sound
D. Dry, nonproductive cough
E. Heart rate of 69 and irregular

HESI Test Question Approach		
Positive?	YES	NO
Key Words		
Rephrase		
Rule Out Choices		
A	B	C	D

Inflammatory Heart Disease
- Endocarditis
  — S/S: fever, murmur, heart failure symptoms (dyspnea, etc.)
  — Infective endocarditis can lead to damaged heart valves
  — Administer antibiotics for 4 to 6 weeks
  — Teach client about anticoagulant therapy
- Pericarditis
  — S/S: pain—hurts more with deep breath, pericardial friction rub
  — Monitor for ST-segment elevation
  — Monitor hemodynamic status
  — *high dose NSAIDS & pain meds*

Handwritten margin notes:
Vegetation on heart valves
— can break off as embolism
deep inspiratory breath leads to chest pain
left lower sternal border is where pericardial rub best heard

Valvular Heart Disease

- Valves may be unable to:
  — Fully open (stenosis)
  — Fully close (insufficiency or regurgitation)
- Causes
  — Rheumatic fever
  — Congenital heart disease
  — Syphilis
  — Endocarditis
  — Hypertension

Mitral Valve Stenosis

- Early period—may have no symptoms
- Later—excessive fatigue, dyspnea on exertion, orthopnea, dry cough, hemoptysis, or pulmonary edema
- Rumbling apical diastolic murmur and atrial fibrillation are common

Nursing and Collaborative Management

See section on heart failure.

- Monitor for a-fib with thrombus formation
- Give prophylactic antibiotic therapy before any invasive procedures (dental, surgical, childbirth)
- May require surgical repair or valve replacement
- With valve replacement: teach client about need for lifelong anticoagulant therapy

The nurse receives report on four clients on the cardiac unit. Which client should the nurse assess first?

A. The client with thrombophlebitis and a positive Homans sign

B. The client with left-sided heart failure and an S3 gallop

C. The client with pericarditis and inspiratory chest pain

D. The client with halo vision after digitalization

[handwritten: indication of dig. toxicity]

[handwritten right margin: Mechanical Valve — anticoagulants for remainder of life]

HESI Test Question Approach			
Positive?		YES	NO
Key Words			
Rephrase			
Rule Out Choices			
A	B	C	D

[handwritten below table: expected findings]

Vascular Disorders
Arterial

- Smooth, shiny skin
- Pallor on elevation
- Weak peripheral pulses
- Sharp or tingling pain
- Cool to touch
- Intermittent claudication (classic symptom)
- Painful, nonedematous ulcers

Venous

- Monitor for history of deep vein thrombosis
- Bluish purple skin discoloration

- Normal peripheral pulses
- Warm to touch
- Slightly painful ulcers with marked edema

Nursing and Collaborative Management

General

- Change positions frequently; avoid sitting with crossed legs
- Wear *no* restrictive clothing
- Keep extremities warm with clothing, not external heaters
- Discourage smoking
- With thrombosis: administer thrombolytic agents

Arterial

- Bed rest
- Topical antibiotics
- Surgical intervention

Abdominal Aortic Aneurysm

- Pulsating abdominal mass
- Bruit heard over abdomen
- Confirmed on radiograph
- With rupture: S/S of hypovolemic shock
- Postoperative care after surgical repair of aneurysm
  — Monitor for S/S of renal failure, postoperative ileus
  — Changes in pulses, S/S of occluded graft

Venous Thromboembolism (VTE)

- Inflammation of the venous wall with clot formation
- S/S: calf pain, edema of calf, induration (hardening) along the blood vessel warmth and redness
  NOTE: Pain in the calf on dorsiflexion of the foot (+ Homans sign) appears in only a small percentage of clients with DVT, and false-positive findings are common. Therefore, relying on a Homans sign is not advised.
- Restrict ambulation
- Elevate extremity
- Antiembolic stockings
- Medications
  — Heparin therapy
    • Therapeutic levels of aPTTs are usually 1 ½ to 2 times normal control levels
    • Protamine sulfate antidote
  — Coumadin therapy
    • Monitor prothrombin time (PT), international normalized ratio (INR)
    • Vitamin K: antidote
  — Antiplatelet agents
    • Ticlopidine (Ticlid)
    • Clopidogrel bisulfate (Plavix)

Which client should the nurse assess first?

A. The client receiving oxygen per nasal cannula who is dyspneic on mild exertion and has a hemoglobin of 70 mmol/L (7 g/dL)

B. The client receiving IV aminoglycosides per CVC who complains of nausea and has a trough level below therapeutic levels

C. The client receiving packed RBCs who complains of flank pain and has a BP of 98/52 mmHg *(indicates rx)*

D. The client receiving chemotherapy whose temperature is 37.2° C (98.9° F) and who has a WBC count of 2.5 × 10^9/L (2,500/mm³)

HESI Test Question Approach		
Positive?	**YES**	**NO**
Key Words		
Rephrase		
Rule Out Choices		
A	B	C	D

Interpret the rhythm

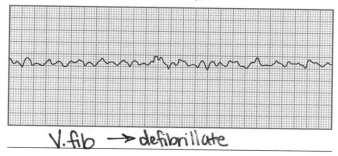

V. fib → defibrillate

(From Urden L et al: *Critical care nursing: diagnosis and management,* ed 6, p 394, St Louis, 2010, Mosby.)

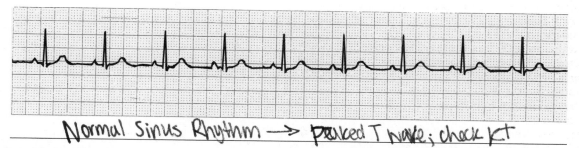

Normal Sinus Rhythm → Peaked T wave; check K+

(From Sole M: *Introduction to critical care nursing,* ed 6, p 112, Philadelphia, 2013, Saunders.)

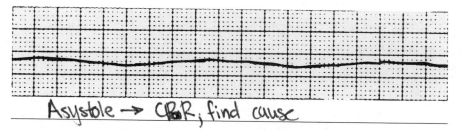

Asystole → CPR; find cause

(In Sole M et al: *Introduction to critical care nursing,* ed 6, p 128, Philadelphia, 2013, Saunders.)

The nurse is ordering afternoon snacks for several clients. Which client will benefit from a snack of cheese-and-bacon scrambled eggs with added protein powder?

A. The client with cirrhosis
B. The client with paralytic ileus
C. The client with cholelithiasis
D. The client with dumping syndrome

benefits from high fat, high protein diet

HESI Test Question Approach		
Positive?	YES	NO
Key Words		
Rephrase		
Rule Out Choices		
A̶	B̶	C̶	D

limited protein   NPO   gallbladder

Gastroesophageal Reflux Disease (GERD)

- Not a disease but a syndrome
- Any clinically significant symptomatic condition secondary to reflux of gastric contents into the lower esophagus
- Most common upper GI problem seen in adults

Etiology and Pathophysiology

There is no single cause of GERD. Predisposing conditions include:

- Hiatal hernia
- Incompetent lower esophageal sphincter (LES)
- Decreased esophageal clearance (ability to clear liquids or food from the esophagus into the stomach) resulting from impaired esophageal motility
- Decreased gastric emptying

Nursing Assessment

- Heartburn after eating
- Fullness and discomfort after eating
- Ask client what foods seem to aggravate symptoms
- Positive diagnosis from barium swallow or fluoroscopy (hiatal hernia)

Nursing Plans and Interventions

- Encourage small frequent meals
- Sit up while eating and remain upright for 1 hour after eating
- Stop eating 3 hours before bedtime
- Elevate head of bed with 4- to 6-inch blocks

Peptic Ulcer Disease
- Significant gastric ulcers are caused by *Helicobacter pylori* bacteria
- Risk factors
  - Drugs: NSAIDs, corticosteroids
  - Alcohol
  - Cigarette smoking
  - Trauma

[handwritten: bleeding is a concern. Most often duodenal]

Nursing Assessment
- Left epigastric pain, may radiate to back
- Epigastric pain relieved with food
- Diagnosis
  - Barium swallow
  - Upper endoscopy

Nursing Plans and Interventions
- Onset of symptoms
- What relieves symptoms *[handwritten: → food/eating]*
- Monitor stools for color, consistency, occult blood
- Administer antacids and antibiotics as ordered
- Avoid caffeine
- Small, frequent meals are best

[handwritten: PPI for patients w/ musculoskeletal issues for prophylaxis]

Complications
- Uncontrolled bleeding
  - Prepare for immediate surgery
- Dumping syndrome—postoperative complication
  - Occurs 5 to 30 minutes after eating
  - Vertigo, syncope, tachycardia
  - Small, frequent meals
  - High-fat, high-protein, low-CHO diet
  - Avoid liquids with meals

Client Teaching
- Avoid certain medications
  - Salicylates
  - NSAIDs
- Inform healthcare personnel of history of peptic ulcer disease
- Symptoms of GI bleeding
  - Dark, tarry stools
  - Coffee ground emesis
  - Bright red rectal bleeding

[handwritten: Dumping Syndrome: low carbs, avoid liquids when eating]

Crohn's Disease (Regional Enteritis)
- Affects both small and large intestines
- Inflammation extends through all layers of intestine
- Right lower quadrant abdominal pain *[handwritten: ; not relieved w/ defecation]*
- Nausea and vomiting
- 3 to 4 stools per day
- Barium enema shows narrowing with areas of stricture separated by segments of normal bowels.
- Capsule endoscopy has shown greater sensitivity than radiography for diagnosis

[handwritten: Targets two periods of life - young & old]

Nursing and Collaborative Management

- Initial treatment is based on symptomatic relief, which usually includes parenteral replacement of fluids, electrolytes, and blood products. Complete bed rest and assistance with ADL during acute phases are prescribed.

Pharmacotherapy

- Sedatives and tranquilizers—to promote rest and reduce anxiety
- Antidiarrheal medications—to reduce diarrhea and cramping
- Sulfasalazine (Salazopyrin [Canada], Azulfidine, Azulfidine EN-tabs)—to treat acute exacerbations of colonic and ileocolonic disease
- Corticosteroids (prednisone [Winpred])—to reduce the active inflammatory response
- Immunosuppressive agents (infliximab [Remicade], adalimumab [Humira])—to allow dosage reduction or withdrawal of corticosteroids.
- Antibiotics—to control infections and perianal fistulas

Nutritional Management

- During acute exacerbations: TPN and NPO (bowel rest)
- Elemental diet
- Bland diets
- No milk, milk products
- Supplementation of vitamins and minerals, especially calcium, iron, folate, magnesium, vitamin D

Surgical Management

- Surgical management is reserved for complications rather than used as a primary form of therapy. Common indications for surgery include bowel obstruction, internal and enterocutaneous fistulas, intraabdominal abscesses, and perianal disease.

Ulcerative Colitis

- Occurs in the large bowel and rectum
- Sigmoidoscopy and colonoscopy allow direct examination of the large intestinal mucosa and are used for diagnosis
- Symptoms
  — Diarrhea
  — Abdominal pain
  — Liquid stools—10 to 20/day
  — Anemia

Nursing Interventions

- Low-residue, low-fat, high-protein, high-calorie diet
- No dairy products
- Tepid fluids
- Daily calorie count
- Monitor I & O

Handwritten notes:

Monitor H&H

given during exacerbations

Inflammation in GI tract:
NPO
~~NG tube~~ IVF
~~PO~~ NG Tube
...
bland diet
back to base

Low residue diet
7 to 10g fiber
avoid peels
low fat, high protein
no dairy
To decrease GI activity

; blood in stool
Monitor H&H for anemia

Tenestenous

- Medications
  — Corticosteroids
  — Antidiarrheals
  — Sulfasalazine (Salazopyrin [Canada], Azulfidine)
  — Infliximab (Remicade) or other biological treatments

Diverticular Diseases
- Left lower quadrant pain
- S/S of intestinal obstruction
  — Abdominal distention
  — Constipation/diarrhea/*Vomiting*
- + Barium enema
- Colonoscopy

High Pitched bowel sounds initially, then absent

Nursing and Collaborative Management
- High-fiber diet unless inflammation is present
- If inflammation is present:
  — NPO
  — Then low-residue, bland diet
  — Bulk-forming laxatives
  — Avoid heavy lifting, tight clothing, and straining
  — *no foods w/ seeds*

NPO
IVF
NG Tube

Intestinal Obstruction
- Mechanical causes
  — Adhesions most common
  — Strangulated hernia
  — Tumors
- Neurogenic causes
  — Paralytic ileus
  — Spinal cord lesion
- Vascular cause
  — Mesenteric artery occlusion

Nursing Assessment
- Sudden abdominal pain
- History of obstruction
- High-pitched bowel sounds (early mechanical obstruction)
- Bowel sounds diminished or absent (neurogenic or late mechanical obstruction)

Nursing and Collaborative Management
- NPO
- IV fluids
- Nasogastric tube to intermittent suction

Liver, Pancreas, and Biliary Tract Problems

A client is receiving pancreatic enzyme replacement therapy for chronic pancreatitis. Which statement by the client indicates a need for more effective teaching?
A. "I will need to mix the enzyme with a protein food."
B. "I will take the enzymes with each meal."
C. "My stools will decrease in number and frequency."
D. "My abdominal pain may lessen."

Protein can de-activate the enzymes.

HESI Test Question Approach		
Positive?	YES	NO
Key Words		
Rephrase		
Rule Out Choices		
A	B	C	D

The nurse is providing discharge instructions to a client after a colon resection. Which statement by the client indicates that teaching has been effective?
A. "It is normal for the incision site to be warm."
B. "I will take my pain medications around the clock."
C. "I will call the healthcare provider if my temperature goes above 38° C (100.4° F)."
D. "I will resume sexual activity this week."

A temp may indicate infection.

HESI Test Question Approach		
Positive?	YES	NO
Key Words		
Rephrase		
Rule Out Choices		
A	B	C	D

Cirrhosis
- Degeneration of the liver tissue
- Chronic progressive disease

Nursing Assessment
- Early sign: RUQ pain
- History
  — ETOH abuse
  — Street and prescriptive drug abuse
  — Exposure to hepatotoxins
  — Jaundice
- Dark-colored urine
- Clay-colored stools
- Yellow sclera
- Fruity or musty breath *(fetor hepaticus)* → *buildup of amino acid*
- Asterixis
- Palmar erythema
- Ascites
- Weight loss

Esophageal Varices
- A common complication of cirrhosis; may rupture and cause hemorrhage

Ammonia buildup leads to confusion → lactulose

Treatment

- Esophagogastric balloon
- Blakemore-Sengstaken tube
- Vitamin K
- Blood products
- Coagulation factors

See Table 6.1 in Appendix B

Nursing and Collaborative Management

- Monitor for bleeding
  — Avoid injections
  — Maintain pressure for 5 minutes after venipunctures
- Provide skin care
  — Avoid soap
  — Apply lotions
- Monitor fluid and electrolytes/ascites
  — Accurate I & O
  — Weigh daily
  — Restrict fluids (1,500 mL/day)
  — Abdominal girth
  — Prepare for paracentesis and peritoneovenous shunts

Dietary Teaching

- May need to restrict protein
- Low sodium
- Low potassium
- Low fat
- High carbohydrate
- May need to take lactulose (Cephulac) as ammonia detoxicant/stimulant laxative

Hepatitis

Widespread inflammation of liver cells, usually caused by a virus

Nursing Assessment

- Risk groups
  — Homosexual males
  — IV drug users (disease is transmitted by contaminated needles)
  — Tattoo/body piercing with contaminated needles;
  — Those living in crowded conditions
  — Healthcare workers employed in high-risk areas
- Fatigue, weakness
- Anorexia, nausea
- Jaundice
- Dark urine
- Joint pain, muscle aches
- Elevated liver enzymes (ALT, AST, alkaline phosphatase), bilirubin

Nursing and Collaborative Management

- Frequent rest periods
- Provide high-calorie, high-carbohydrate diet with moderate fats and proteins
- Administer antiemetic as needed
- Avoid alcohol intake and drugs detoxified by the liver

Pancreatitis

- Acute: autodigestion of the pancreas
  — Alcohol ingestion and biliary tract disease are major causes.
- Chronic: progressive, destructive disease
  — Long-term alcohol use is a major factor in disease.

Pancreatic Enzymes: lypase, amylase, tripsin

Acute Pancreatitis Assessment

Abdominal pain is the predominant symptom of acute pancreatitis.

- Located in the left upper quadrant
- Radiates to the back
- Sudden onset
- Described as severe, deep, piercing, and continuous
- Aggravated by eating and is not relieved by vomiting
- Accompanied by flushing, cyanosis, and dyspnea

Other Manifestations of Acute Pancreatitis

- Nausea and vomiting
- Low-grade fever
- Leukocytosis
- Jaundice
- Abdominal tenderness with muscle guarding
- Bowel sounds may be decreased or absent, and ileus may occur
- Areas of ecchymoses *Grey Turner's spots* or *sign,* a bluish flank discoloration and *Cullen's sign,* a bluish periumbilical discoloration
- Hypotension
- Tachycardia
- Hypovolemia (massive fluid shift into the retroperitoneal space)
- Shock (hemorrhage into the pancreas)
- Toxemia (activated pancreatic enzymes)
- Lungs frequently involved (crackles)

Chronic Pancreatitis Assessment

- Steatorrhea
- Diarrhea
- Jaundice
- Ascites
- Weight loss

— due to long term alcohol abuse

Nursing Plans and Interventions

- Acute management
  — NPO
  — NG tube to suction
  — Morphine or hydromorphone (Dilaudid) are typically used for pain management
  — Sitting up or leaning forward may reduce pain
  — Monitor blood sugar
  — Teach foods and fluids to avoid

- Chronic management
  — Pain management
    - Morphine
  — Pancreatic enzymes
    - Mix powdered forms with fruit juice or applesauce; avoid mixing with proteins
  — Histamine blocker agents
    - Teach foods and fluids to avoid

A client who has an obstruction of the common bile duct caused by cholelithiasis passes clay-colored stools containing streaks of fat. What action should the nurse take?
A. Auscultate for diminished bowel sounds
B. Send a stool specimen to the lab
C. Document the assessment in the chart
D. Notify the healthcare provider

expected finding

HESI Test Question Approach			
Positive?		YES	NO
Key Words			
Rephrase			
Rule Out Choices			
A	B	C	D

Cholecystitis and Cholelithiasis
- Cholecystitis: acute inflammation of the gallbladder
- Cholelithiasis: formation or presence of gallstones

Nursing Assessment
- Pain
- Fever
- Elevated WBCs
- Abdominal tenderness
- Jaundice

Nursing Plans and Interventions
- Analgesics for pain
- NPO
- NG to suction
- IV antibiotics
- Low-fat diet
  — Avoid fried, spicy, and fatty foods

Treatment
- Cholecystitis
  — IV hydration
  — Administer antibiotics
  — Pain management
- Cholelithiasis (gallstones)
  — Nonsurgical removal
    - Endoscopic retrograde cholangiopancreatography (ERCP)
    - Lithotripsy
  — Surgical approach
    - Cholecystectomy, laparoscopic or open

A client is admitted with gastric ulcer disease and GI bleeding. Which risk factor should the nurse identify in the client's history?

A. Eats heavily seasoned foods
B. Uses NSAIDs daily
C. Consumes alcohol every day
D. Follows an acid-ash diet

(meat, eggs, cheese; used to acidify the urine)

HESI Test Question Approach

Positive?		YES	NO
Key Words	risk factor		
Rephrase			
Rule Out Choices			
~~A~~	B	~~C~~	D

irritants

The nurse is caring for a client with peritonitis. Which information should the nurse report immediately to the healthcare provider?

A. Blood pressure readings of 92/64, 110/70, and 100/68 over the past hour
B. Urine output of 300 mL over the past 8 hours
C. Rebound tenderness, and pain the client rates as a 7 on a 0 to 10 scale
D. Dry mucous membranes and nausea

may indicate perforation

HESI Test Question Approach

Positive?		YES	NO
Key Words			
Rephrase			
Rule Out Choices			
A	B	C	D

Renal and Urological Problems

Urinary Tract Infections

- Obtain clean-catch midstream specimen
- Administer antibiotics as ordered
  — Take fully prescribed dose
  — Do not skip doses
- Encourage fluid intake of 3,000 mL/day
- Encourage voiding every 2 to 3 hours

Urinary Tract Obstruction

- Caused by calculi or stones
- Location of pain can help locate stone
  — Flank pain (stone usually in upper ureter)
  — Pain radiating to abdomen (stone likely in ureter or bladder)

Nursing Interventions

- Administer narcotics   *pain management!*
- Strain all urine
- Encourage high fluid intake
  — 3 to 4 L/day
- Strict I & O ; *strain urine to catch stone*
- May need surgical management

Benign Prostatic Hyperplasia

- Enlargement of the prostrate
  — Most common treatment: transurethral resection of the prostate (TURP)
  — Can be done with laser to burn out prostate
  — If prostate is too large, suprapubic approach is used
- Assess for:
  — Increased urinary frequency/decreased output
  — Bladder distention (increases risk of spasm)

Nursing Plans and Interventions

- Preoperative teaching
  — Pain management
  — Oversized balloon catheter
- Bladder spasms
  — Common after surgery
  — Use antispasmodics
    • Belladonna and opium suppositories
    • Oxybutynin chloride (Ditropan)
    • Dicyclomine hydrochloride (Bentylol)
- Continuous bladder irrigation is typically done to remove blood clots and ensure drainage.
- Drainage should be reddish pink for 24 hours, clearing to light pink.
- Monitor color and amount of urine output.
- Notify physician if client has bright red bleeding with large clots.

Discharge Teaching

- Continue to drink 12 to 14 glasses of water per day
- Avoid straining
- Avoid strenuous activity, sports, lifting, and intercourse for 3 to 4 weeks
- Report large amounts of blood or frank blood

The charge nurse is making assignments on the renal unit. Which client should the nurse assign to a PN who is new to the unit?

A. An older client who has thick, dark red drainage in a urinary catheter 1 day after a transurethral prostatic resection
B. A middle-aged client admitted with acute renal failure secondary to a reaction to IVP dye
C. An older client who has end-stage renal disease and who complains of nausea after receiving digoxin
D. A middle-aged client who receives hemodialysis and has been prescribed epoetin alfa subcutaneous daily

[handwritten: bladder irrigation]
[handwritten: Monitor for clots/bloody urine]

[handwritten: Scope of practice / Stability of patient]
[handwritten: Stimulates red blood cell production]

HESI Test Question Approach			
Positive?		**YES**	**NO**
Key Words	new to unit		
Rephrase			
Rule Out Choices			
A	B	C	D

A client who was admitted for acute renal failure has a potassium level of <u>6.4 mmol/L</u> (mEq/L). Which snack should the nurse offer?

A. An orange
B. A milkshake → *milk products contain k⁺*
C. Dried fruit and nuts
D. A gelatin dessert

little to no k⁺

Acute Renal Failure (ARF)

- A reversible syndrome if symptoms are caught early enough
- Remember:
  — Kidneys use 25% of normal cardiac output to maintain function.
  — Kidneys excrete 1 to 2 L of urine per 24 hours for adults.
  — Three types of ARF:
    - Prerenal
    - Intrarenal
    - Postrenal

30cc/hr

Prerenal Failure

- Etiological factors
  — Hemorrhage
  — Hypovolemia
  — Decreased cardiac output
  — Decreased renal perfusion

Intrarenal Failure

- Etiological factors
  — May develop secondary to prerenal failure
  — Nephrotoxins
  — Infections (glomerulonephritis)
  — Renal injury
  — Vascular lesions

Postrenal Failure

- Etiological factors for obstruction
  — Calculi
  — Benign prostatic hyperplasia (BPH)
  — Tumors
  — Strictures

prerenal — before kidney
intrarenal — within kidney
postrenal — between kidney & bladder

Nursing Assessment

- Decreased urine output
- Weight gain
- Edema
- Diagnostic test results—oliguric phase
  — ↓ Urine output
  — ↑ BUN (blood urea nitrogen) and creatinine
  — ↑ Potassium
  — ↓ Sodium (serum)
  — ↓ pH
  — Metabolic acidosis
  — ↑ Urine sodium
  — Fixed at 1.010 specific gravity
- Diagnostic test results—diuretic phase
  — ↑ Urine output
  — ↓ Fluid volume
  — ↓ Potassium
  — ↓ Sodium
  — ↓ Urine specific gravity
  — ↓ Urine sodium

→ very little urine

→ up to 10,000 cc/24hr

Nursing Plans and Interventions

- Oliguric phase: Give only enough fluids to replace losses + 400 to 500 mL/24 hr
- Strict I & O
- Monitor lab values closely
- Watch for ECG changes
- Monitor weight daily

1:1 fluids (in) (out)

After hemodialysis, the nurse is evaluating the blood results for a client who has end-stage renal disease. Which value should the nurse verify with the laboratory?
- A. Elevated serum potassium
- B. Increase in serum calcium
- C. Low hemoglobin
- D. Reduction in serum sodium

hyperkalemia should be corrected by dialysis

HESI Test Question Approach			
Positive?		YES	NO
Key Words	very	verify	
	hemodialysis		
Rephrase			
Rule Out Choices			
A	B	C	D

Chronic Kidney Disease (CKD)

- End-stage renal disease
- Progressive irreversible damage to the nephrons and glomeruli
- Causes
  — Diabetic nephropathy
  — Hypertensive nephrosclerosis
  — Glomerulonephritis
  — Polycystic kidney disease

Nursing Assessment

- Early stage
  - Polyuria
  - Renal insufficiency
- Late stage
  - Oliguria
  - Hematuria
  - Proteinuria
  - Edema
  - Increased BP
  - Muscle wasting secondary to negative nitrogen balance
  - Ammonia taste in mouth
  - ↑ Creatinine, ↑ phosphorus, ↑ potassium
- End stage
  - Anuria (<100 mL/24 hr)

Nursing and Collaborative Management

- Monitor serum electrolytes
- Weigh daily
- Strict I & O
- Renal diet
  - Low protein → *guided by GFR*
  - Low sodium
  - Low potassium
  - Low phosphate

Medications

- Drugs are used to manage associated complications.
  - **Aluminum hydroxide** (to bind phosphates) → *give w/ food*
  - **Epoetin** (Eprex [Canada], Epogen) (to treat anemia)
  - **Antihypertensive therapy**
  - **Calcium supplements** and **vitamin D**
  - **Antihyperlipidemics**
  - **Statins** (to lower LDL)
  - **Fibrates** (to lower triglycerides)
- CAUTION: As kidney function decreases, medication doses need adjustment.

Renal Dialysis

- Hemodialysis
  - AV fistula → *check for thrill & bruit*
- Ø Venipunctures, Ø IVs, Ø BP in AV shunt arm
- Withhold medications that would affect hemodynamic stability before dialysis
- Peritoneal dialysis
  - Monitor indwell and outflow times closely
  - Monitor I & O

Postoperative Care: Kidney Surgery

- Respiratory status
  - Auscultate to detect rales or rhonchi
  - Demonstrate splinting method
- Circulatory status
  - Monitor for shock
  - Monitor surgical site for bleeding
- Pain relief status
  - Administer narcotic analgesics as needed

76

- Urinary status
  — Check urinary output and drainage from *all* tubes
  — Strict I & O

A client with a 20-year history of type 1 diabetes mellitus is having renal function tests because of recent fatigue, weakness, a blood urea nitrogen (BUN) of 8.5 mmol/L (24 mg/dL), and a serum creatinine of 146 mcmol/L (1.6 mg/dL). What other early symptom of renal insufficiency might the nurse expect?

A. Dyspnea
B. Nocturia
C. Confusion
D. Stomatitis

HESI Test Question Approach			
Positive?		YES	NO
Key Words			
Rephrase			
Rule Out Choices			
A	B	C	D

7 Regulatory, Reproductive, and Urinary

A male client who has type 1 diabetes returns to the clinic for follow-up after dietary counseling. The client states that he has been managing his diabetes very closely. Which lab result indicates that the client is maintaining tight control of the disease?

A. FBS changes from 7.5 to 6 mmol/L (135 to 110 mg/dL)
B. SMBG at bedtime changes from 2.5 to 5 mmol/L (45 to 90 mg/dL)
C. Glycosylated hemoglobin (Hemoglobin A1c) changes from 9% to 6%   *<7% ideal*
D. Urine ketones change from 0 to 3

best indicator of long term control of diabetes

A 36-year-old married male with a BMI of 33 declares that he wants to lose weight. In addition to dietary intake and level of physical activity, what data are most necessary for the nurse to collect before planning care?

A. Draw blood for determination of a resting metabolic rate
B. Determine who prepares the meals *& who buys food*
C. Identify the client's educational level
D. Ascertain the client's smoking history

Obesity, Metabolic Syndrome, Prediabetes, and Diabetes

- **Primary obesity** develops when the calorie intake exceeds the body's metabolic needs.
- Assessed by using a body mass index (BMI) chart.
  - BMI of 18.5 to 24.9 kg/m^2: Normal weight
  - BMI of 25 to 29.9 kg/m^2: Overweight
  - BMI $\geq$ 30 kg/m^2 : Obese
  - BMI > 40 kg/m^2: Morbidly obese
- Abdominal and visceral fat have been linked to metabolic syndrome.
- Disproportionally represented in minority populations

Assessment
- Risk factor screening
  - Cardiovascular disease
  - Hypertension
  - Sleep apnea
  - Type 2 diabetes
  - Osteoporosis
  - Motivational interviewing

Nursing and Collaborative Management
- Life style management
  - Medical nutritional therapy
  - Physical activity
  - Behavior modification
- Pharmacological therapy
- Bariatric surgery
  - Criteria for bariatric surgery include a BMI $\geq$ 40 kg/m^2 or a BMI $\geq$ 35 kg/m^2 with one or more severe, obesity-related medical complications
  - Gastric bypass, gastric banding, Roux-en-Y

Metabolic syndrome is a collection of risk factors that increase an individual's chance of developing cardiovascular disease and diabetes mellitus.

Assessment
- Meets three or more criteria:
  - **Waist circumference** $\geq$ 40 inches (102 cm) in men or $\geq$ 35 inches (88 cm) in women
  - **Triglycerides** > 1.81 mmol/L (160 mg/dL) or drug treatment for elevated triglycerides
  - **High-density lipoprotein (HDL) cholesterol** < 1.036 mmol/L (40 mg/dL in men or < 50 mg/dL in women); or, drug treatment for reduced HDL cholesterol
  - **BP** $\geq$ 130 mmHg systolic or $\geq$ 85 mmHg diastolic; or, drug treatment for hypertension
  - **Fasting blood glucose level** $\geq$ 6 mmol/L (110 mg/dL) or drug treatment for elevated glucose level

Nursing and Collaborative Management
- Lifestyle management:
  - Medical nutritional therapy
  - Physical activity
  - Behavior modification

Prediabetes is a condition in which individuals are at increased risk for developing diabetes. In this condition, the blood glucose levels are high but not high enough to meet the diagnostic criteria for diabetes.

Assessment
- Fasting blood glucose level: 5.6–6.9 mmol/L (100-125 mg/dL)
- 2-hour oral glucose tolerance test (OGTT) values: < 7.8 mmol/L (< 140 mg/dL)
- Glycosylated hemoglobin (Hemoglobin A1c): 5.7% to 6.4%

Nursing and Collaborative Management
- Lifestyle management:
  - Medical nutritional therapy
  - Physical activity
  - Behavior modification

Diabetes mellitus is a chronic multisystem disease related to abnormal insulin production, impaired insulin use, or both.
  - *Type 1 diabetes:* Immune-mediated disease associated with absolute insulin deficiency. The body's own T cells destroy pancreatic beta cells, which are the source of insulin.

— *Type 2 diabetes:* The defect is insulin resistance and relative insulin deficiency. There is insufficient insulin production, insulin resistance, and/or excessive and unregulated glucose production from the liver.
— Other types of diabetes
  • Cystic fibrosis related diabetes
  • Transplant related diabetes
  • Gestational diabetes
  • Steroid induced diabetes
  • Hospital related hyperglycemia

Clinical Manifestations

■ Type 1

[handwritten: excess urine ↑ ... eating ↑ ... drinking ↓]

— Abrupt onset of polyuria, polydipsia, polyphagia and weight loss
— Weakness and fatigue
— Ketoacidosis may occur
  • Serum glucose ≥ 13.9 mmol/L (250 mg/dL); ketonuria in large amounts
  • Arterial pH of < 7.30 and HCO_3 < 15 mmol/L (mEq/L)
  • Serum bicarbonate < 15 mmol/L (mEq/dL), nausea, vomiting, dehydration, abdominal pain, Kussmaul's respirations, acetone odor to breath
— Onset typically in childhood or adolescence but can occur at any age
■ Type 2
— Risk factors
  • Age ≥45 years
  • Overweight (BMI > 25)
  • First-degree relative with diabetes
  • Sedentary lifestyle
  • Ethnic at-risk group
  • Gestational diabetes or a baby > 9 lb
  • CVD and/ or hypertension
  • Abnormal lipids (low HDL, high TG)
  • Previous IGT or IFG (prediabetes)
  • PCOS
  • Signs of insulin resistance (acanthosis nigricans)
  • History of CV disease
— Onset is insidious with polyuria, polyphagia, polydipsia, and weight loss. Client may experience fatigue, recurrent infections, prolonged wound healing, blurred vision, and impotence.
— Rare development of ketoacidosis. Client is more likely to develop hyperosmolar hyperglycemia nonketotic syndrome (HHNKS) with blood sugars > 33.3 mmol/L (600 mg/dL).
— Plasma hyperosmolality
— Dehydration
— Altered mental status
— Absent ketone bodies

Diagnosis

A1c ≥ 6.5% or FPG ≥126 mg/dL or 2-h plasma glucose ≥ 200 mg/dL or classic symptoms + random plasma glucose ≥ 200 mg/dL. Results should be confirmed by repeat testing

[handwritten right column:]

$\frac{20}{200}$ = legal blindness

$\frac{160}{20}$ = farsightedness

$\frac{20}{60}$ = nearsightedness
indicator of retinopathy
(diabetic complication)

Assessment

- Integument: Skin breakdown
- Eyes: Retinal problems, cataracts
- Kidneys: Edema, urinary retention
- Periphery: Cool skin, numbness, tingling
- Ulcerations on extremities and thick nails
- Cardiopulmonary angina and dyspnea

Nursing and Collaborative Management

- Medical nutrition therapy
  - Type 1: Integrate insulin with eating and exercise
  - Type 2: Heart-healthy diet and moderate weight loss of 10% to 20%
    - 55% to 60% carbohydrate
    - 12% to 15% protein
    - 30% fat
    - Space meals
    - Regular activity
- Monitoring
  - Detects extremes and targets
  - Educate client in techniques, calibration, and record keeping   *→ check feet for wounds*
- Physical activity
  - Moderate-intensity aerobic physical activity, 150 minutes per week; resistance training, 3 days per week
- Education
  - Medication management including injection techniques if injectable prescribed
  - Monitor for S/S of hypoglycemia/hyperglycemia
  - Foot care
  - Manage sick days
    - Keep taking insulin
    - Check blood sugar more frequently
    - Watch for S/S of hyperglycemia

The RN assigns the PN a client with diabetes. Which findings should the RN instruct the PN to report immediately?

A. Fingerstick blood glucose level of 13.7 mmol/L (247 mg/dL)
B. Diaphoresis and headache
C. Crackles at the end of inspiration
D. Numbness in the fingertips and toes

Correlates w/ hypoglycemia

Pharmacological Intervention
Oral Agents and Injectables

- Key principles
  - Oral agents are not insulin; they work on the three defects of type 2 diabetes:
    - Insulin resistance
    - Decreased insulin production
    - Increased hepatic glucose production

HESI Test Question Approach			
Positive?		**YES**	**NO**
Key Words			
Rephrase			
Rule Out Choices			
A	B	C	D

- **Sulfonylureas:** Increase insulin production from the pancreas; therefore, hypoglycemia is the major side effect.
  - Glipizide (Glucotrol, Glucotrol XL)
  - Glyburide (DiaBeta, Euglucon)
  - Glimepiride (Amaryl)
  - Gliclazide (Diamicron)
- **Meglitinides:** Increase insulin production from the pancreas. They are short acting and more rapidly absorbed and eliminated than sulfonylureas; therefore, hypoglycemia is a risk. Make sure client has a meal with each dose.
  - Repaglinide (GlucoNorm [Canada], Prandin)
  - Nateglinide (Starlix)
- **Biguanides:** Reduce glucose production by the liver and enhance insulin sensitivity at the tissue level. These are the first-choice drug for most people with type 2 diabetes. Do not use in clients with kidney disease, liver disease, or heart failure or for clients who drink excessive amounts of alcohol.
  - Metformin hydrochloride (Glucophage)
- **α-Glucosidase inhibitors** (starch blockers): Slow the absorption of carbohydrate in the small intestine. Flatus is a common side effect.
  - Acarbose (Glucobay [Canada], Precose)
- **Thiazolidinediones** (insulin sensitizers): Most effective for clients with insulin resistance; do not cause hypoglycemia when used alone.
  - Pioglitazone (Actos)
  - Rosiglitazone (Avandia)
    - Do not use in clients with heart failure because of increased risk of myocardial infarction and stroke
- **Dipeptidyl peptidase-4 (DPP-4) inhibitor:** Inhibits DPP-4, thus slowing the inactivation of incretin hormones. Because the DPP-4 inhibitors are glucose dependent, they lower the potential for hypoglycemia.
  - Sitagliptin (Januvia)
  - Saxagliptin (Onglyza)
- **Incretin mimetic:** Simulate one of the incretin hormones found to be decreased in people with type 2 diabetes. A prefilled pen is used to administer the drug subcutaneously. Acute pancreatitis and kidney problems have been associated with the use of these drugs.
  - Exenatide (Byetta)
  - Liraglutide (Victoza)
- **Amylin analog:** A synthetic analog of human amylin; indicated for clients with type 1 diabetes and for those with type 2 diabetes who have not achieved glucose control despite the use of insulin at mealtimes. This drug is administered subcutaneously and cannot be mixed with insulin; severe hypoglycemia can result if the drug is used with insulin.
  - Pramlintide (Symlin)

Do not use oral prior to surgery or during pregnancy.

Insulin Pharmacokinetics after Subcutaneous Injection

- **Rapid-acting insulin:** Can be given IV
  - Glulisine (Apidra)—given within 15 minutes of meal
    - Onset: 0.25 hr
    - Peak: 1 hr
    - Duration: 2-3 hr
  - Lispro (Humalog)—given within 15 minutes of meal
    - Onset: 0.25 hr
    - Peak: 1 hr
    - Duration: 4 hr
  - Aspart (NovoRapid [Canada], NovoLog)—given within 15 minutes of meal
    - Onset: 0.5 hr
    - Peak: 1-3 hr
    - Duration: 3-5 hr
  - Regular (Humulin R)—given within 30 minutes of meal
    - Onset: 0.5-1 hr
    - Peak: 2-4 hr
    - Duration: 5-7 hr
- **Intermediate-acting insulin:** Do not give IV; can be mixed with rapid-acting insulins (see Combinations section, below).
  - Isophane Insulin suspension NPH, Humulin N)
    - Onset: 3-4 hr
    - Peak: 6-12 hr
    - Duration: 18-28 hr
- **Long-acting insulin:** Cannot be mixed with any other type of insulin. Usually given once a day in the morning. Acts as basal insulin. Do not shake solutions. CAUTION: Solution is clear; do not confuse with regular insulin.
  - Glargine (Lantus)
    - Onset: 1-5 hr
    - Peak: Plateau
    - Duration: 24 hr
  - Detemir (Levemir)
    - Onset: 3-4 hr
    - Peak: Peakless
    - Duration: 24 hr

Combinations (Premix Insulins)

- Regular insulin 30% and NPH 70% (Canada): Humulin 30/70 (Canada); NPH and Regular: (70% NPH insulin and 30% regular insulin)
  - Onset: 0.5-1 hr
  - Peak: 1.5-12 hr
  - Duration: Up to 24 hr
- Lispro insulins: Insulin Lispro protamine suspension 75% and insulin lispro 25% (Humalog Mix 25) (Canada); 75/25 (75% insulin lispro protamine suspension and 25% insulin lispro)
  - Onset: 0.25-0.5 hr
  - Peak: ≥2 hr
  - Duration: Approx. 22 hr

- Lispro: Lisproprotamine suspension 50% and insulin lispro 50% (Humalog Mix 50)(Canada); protamine suspension 50% and insulin lispro 50% (Humalog Mix 50): 50/50 (50% insulin lispro protamine suspension and 50% insulin lispro)
  — Onset: 0.25-0.5 hr
  — Peak: 0.5-1.5 hr
  — Duration: Approx. 22 hr
- Aspart insulins: 30% soluble insulin aspart and 70% insulin aspart protamine crystals (NovoMix 30) (Canada); 70/30 (70% insulin aspart protamine suspension and 30% insulin aspart)
  — Onset: 0.17-0.33 hr
  — Peak: 1-4 hr
  — Duration: Up to 24 hr
- Because analog premixed insulin has a rapid onset, it should be given shortly before meals and should not be given at bedtime. Clients who choose to use premixed insulin preparations should have a fairly routine lifestyle.
- In clients with impaired liver or kidney function, the insulin dosage may need to be reduced, because insulin is metabolized by the liver and excreted by the kidneys.

Other Endocrine Problems

Which client should the nurse assess first?

A. The client with hyperthyroidism exhibiting exophthalmos

B. The client with type 1 diabetes with an inflamed foot ulcer

C. The client with Cushing's syndrome exhibiting moon facies

D. The client with Addison's disease showing tremors and diaphoresis

Addisonian crisis
↳ hypoglycaemia
Monitor glucose and volume

Thyroid Gland Feedback Loop

Hypothalamus
⇩
TRH (+)
Anterior pituitary
— T$_3$ and T$_4$ (−) TSH (+)
— Thyroid gland

Hyperthyroidism
Nursing Assessment
- Enlarged thyroid gland
- Exophthalmos
- Weight loss
- T$_3$ elevated
- T$_4$ elevated

HESI Test Question Approach		
Positive?	**YES**	**NO**
Key Words		
Rephrase		
Rule Out Choices		
A	B	C	D

- Diarrhea
- Tachycardia
- Bruit over thyroid

Nursing Plans and Interventions

- Diet: High protein, high calorie, low caffeine, low fiber
- Treatment may trigger hypothyroidism; client may need hormone replacement.
- Propylthiouracil (PTU) therapy to block the synthesis of T_3 and T_4
- Iodine (^{131}I) therapy to destroy thyroid cells
- Surgical management
  — Thyroidectomy
    - Check behind neck for drainage
    - Support neck when moving client
    - Assess for laryngeal edema
    - Have tracheotomy set, oxygen, and suction equipment at bedside
    - Have calcium gluconate at bedside *Monitor for tetany*

Which adaptation of the environment is most important for the nurse to include in the plan of care for a client with myxedema? *(hypothyroidism)*

A. Reduce environmental stimuli
B. Prevent direct sunlight from entering the room
C. Maintain a warm room temperature
D. Minimize exposure to visitors

Cold intolerance !

Look for bleeding behind the neck first.

HESI Test Question Approach			
Positive?		**YES**	**NO**
Key Words			
Rephrase			
Rule Out Choices			
A	**B**	**C**	**D**

Hypothyroidism

Nursing Assessment

- Fatigue
- Bradycardia
- Weight gain
- Constipation
- Periorbital edema
- Cold intolerance
- Low T_3 (<70)
- Low T_4 (<5)

Nursing Plans and Interventions

- Myxedema coma (acute exacerbation of hypothyroidism)— maintain airway
- Teach medication regimen
- Monitor for side effects of medications
- Monitor bowel program for S/S of constipation

Medications

- **Levothyroxine** Sodium (Eltroxin, Euthyrox, Synthroid)
  — Monitor heart rate
  — Hold for pulse > 100 beats/min
- **Liothyronine** (Cytomel)
  — Increases metabolic rate
  — Acts as synthetic T_3
  — Check hormone levels regularly
  — Avoid food containing iodine
- **Levothyroxine** (T_4) + liothyronine (T_3) (Liotrix)
  — Fast onset

A client is admitted to the hospital with a diagnosis of Addison's crisis. The nurse places a peripheral saline lock. Which prescription should the nurse be prepared to administer?
A. Calcium
B. Glucose
C. Potassium
D. Iodine

hypoglycemia in Addison's crisis

HESI Test Question Approach			
Positive?		YES	NO
Key Words			
Rephrase			
Rule Out Choices			
A	B	C	D

Addison's Disease
Etiology

- Sudden withdrawal from corticosteroids
- Hypofunction of adrenal cortex
- Lack of pituitary ACTH

Signs and Symptoms
Nursing Assessment

- Weight loss
- N/V
- Hypovolemia
- Hypoglycemia
- Hyponatremia
- Hyperkalemia
- Loss of body hair
- Postural hypotension
- Hyperpigmentation

Nursing Plans and Interventions

- Frequent vital signs
- Weigh daily
- Monitor serum electrolytes
- Diet: High sodium, low potassium, high carbohydrates
- Encourage at least 3 L of fluid per day

Maintain low stress environment.

Cushing's Syndrome

Excess adrenocorticoid activity caused by adrenal, pituitary, or hypothalamus tumors

Assessment

- Moon face and edema of lower extremities
- Flat affect
- Obesity

86

- Abdominal striae
- Buffalo hump (fat deposits)
- Muscle atrophy, weakness
- Thin, dry, pale skin
- Hypertension
- Osteoporosis
- Immunosuppressed ▷ *Monitor WBC*
- Hirsutism
- Lab results
  — Hyperglycemia
  — Hypercalcemia
  — Hypernatremia
  — Hypokalemia
  — Increased plasma cortisol levels

Nursing Plans and Interventions
- Monitor for S/S of infection
- Fever
- Skin lesions
- Elevated WBCs
- Diet
  — Low sodium
  — Low carbohydrate

Sexually Transmitted Diseases (STDs)
- Symptoms and treatment
  — Vary by disease
- Teach safer sex
  — Limit number of partners
  — Use latex condoms
- Report incidence of STDs to appropriate health agencies.

Refer to review manuals for more in-depth information about STDs:
- *Evolve Reach Comprehensive Review for the NCLEX-RN Examination (powered by HESI)*
- *Mosby's Comprehensive Review of Nursing for the NCLEX-RN Examination*
- *Saunders Comprehensive Review for the NCLEX-RN Examination*

Female Reproductive Problems

A 52-year-old client who had had an abdominal hysterectomy for cervical adenocarcinoma in situ is preparing for discharge. Which recommendation about women's health and screening examinations should the nurse offer?

A. Continue the annual Pap smear and mammogram, biannual clinical breast examinations, and monthly breast self-examinations (BSE)
B. A Pap smear is no longer necessary, but continue the annual mammogram and biannual clinical breast examinations, plus monthly BSE
C. If the ovaries have been removed, only an annual mammogram and clinical breast examinations are necessary
D. Annual mammograms are not needed if biannual clinical breast examinations and weekly BSE are done

Teaching across the lifespan

HESI Test Question Approach			
Positive?		YES	NO
Key Words			
Rephrase			
Rule Out Choices			
A	B	C	D

Benign Uterine Tumors

- Arise from muscle tissue of the uterus
- Signs and symptoms
  — Menorrhagia
  — Uterine enlargement
  — Dysmenorrhea
  — Anemia secondary to menorrhagia
  — Uterine enlargement
  — Low back pain and pelvic pain
  — Tend to disappear after menopause
- Surgical options
  — Myomectomy *(removal of fibroid)*
  — Hysterectomy
- Fertility issues

After stopping hormone replacement therapy (HRT), a 76-year-old client reports she is experiencing increased vaginal discomfort during intercourse. What action should the nurse take?

A. Suggest the use of a vaginal cream or lubricant
B. Recommend that the client abstain from sexual intercourse
C. Teach the client to perform Kegel exercises daily
D. Instruct the client to resume HRT

vaginal dryness due to lack of estrogen

Uterine Prolapse, Cystocele, and Rectocele

- Preventive measures
  — Postpartum perineal exercises (Kegel)
  — Spaced pregnancy
  — Weight control
- Differing S/S for each condition
- Surgical intervention
  — Hysterectomy
  — Anterior and posterior vaginal repair
- Pain management postoperative
- Monitor urinary output postoperative
- Observe for S/S of postoperative bleeding and infection

A client who had a vaginal hysterectomy the previous day is saturating perineal pads with blood and requires frequent changes during the night. What is the nurse's priority action?

A. Provide iron-rich foods on each dietary tray
B. Monitor the client's vital signs every 2 hours
C. Administer IV fluids at the prescribed rate
D. Encourage postoperative leg exercises

excessive bleeding requires frequent VS w/ BP

HESI Test Question Approach		
Positive?	YES	NO
Key Words		
Rephrase		
Rule Out Choices		
A	B	C	D

HESI Test Question Approach		
Positive?	YES	NO
Key Words		
Rephrase		
Rule Out Choices		
A	B	C	D

Male Reproductive Problems

Etiology and Pathophysiology
Prostatitis is one of the most common urologic disorders.
Common Manifestations (Acute Bacterial Prostatitis)
- Fever
- Chills
- Back pain
- Perineal pain
- Dysuria
- Urinary frequency
- Urgency
- Cloudy urine

Diagnostic Studies
- Urinalysis (UA)
- Urine culture
- White blood cell (WBC) count
- Blood cultures
- PSA test (may be done to rule out prostate cancer)

Management
- Antibiotics
  - Sulfamethoxazole–trimethoprim   (cotrimoxazole) (Bactrim)
  - Ciprofloxacin hydrochloride (Cipro)
  - Ofloxacin (Apo-Ofloxacin [Canada]; Floxin)
  - Doxycycline hyclate (Vibramycin)
  - Tetracycline
- Antiinflammatory agents for pain control

Nursing Intervention
- Encourage fluid intake

Sexual Functioning
- **Vasectomy:** Bilateral surgical ligation of the vas deferens performed for the purpose of sterilization.
- **Erectile dysfunction (ED):** Inability to attain or maintain an erect penis. ED can result from a large number of factors. Causes can include:
  - Diabetes
  - Vascular disease
  - Side effects from medications
  - Result of surgery (prostatectomy)
  - Trauma
  - Chronic illness
  - Decreased gonadal hormone secretion
  - Stress
  - Difficulty in a relationship
  - Depression
  - Vascular disease (the most common cause)

The treatment for ED is based on the underlying cause.

Oral Drug Therapy
- Sildenafil citrate (Viagra)
- Tadalafil (Cialis)
- Vardenafil hydrochloride (Levitra)
- These drugs may potentiate the hypotensive effect of nitrates; they are contraindicated for individuals taking nitrates (e.g., nitroglycerin).

may still be fertile up to one month; need check-ups

8 Movement, Coordination, and Sensory Input

Altered State of Consciousness

- Glasgow Coma Scale
  - Used to assess level of consciousness
  - Maximum score 15, minimum 3
  - Score ≤ 7 = Coma
  - Score 3-4 = High mortality rate
  - Score > 8 = Good prognosis
- Neurological vital signs
  - Pupil size (with sizing scale)
  - Limb movement (with scale)
  - Vital signs (blood pressure, temperature, pulse, respirations)

Table 8-1 Glasgow Coma Scale*

Eye Opening	
Spontaneous	4
To sound	3
To pain	2
Never	1
Motor Response	
Obeys commands	6
Localizes pain	5
Normal flexion (withdrawal)	4
Abnormal flexion	3
Extension	2
None	1
Verbal Response	
Oriented	5
Confused conversation	4
Inappropriate words	3
Incomprehensible sounds	2
None	1

*The highest possible score is 15
Ignatavicius, Workman. *Medical-Surgical Nursing: Patient-Centered Collaborative Care, 7th Edition.* W.B. Saunders Company, 2013.

Nursing Assessment

- Assess for early S/S of changes in level of consciousness (LOC)
  - Decreasing LOC
  - Change in orientation
- Late signs
  - Cushing's triad
    - Widening pulse pressure
    - Slowing heart rate
    - Slowing respirations
  - Change in size, response of pupils, dilated on side of injury initially

— Elevated temperature
- Assess for change in respiratory status
  — Cheyne-Stokes respiration → *rapid breathing w/ pauses*
- Maintain airway—with decreasing LOC will need mechanical ventilation
- Prevent hypoxia
  — Hyperventilate before suctioning
  — Limit suctioning to 15 seconds
    • Keep airway free of secretions
    • Prevent aspiration

Treatment: Increased ICP

- ICP monitoring
  — Goal ICP: <20 mmHg   *720 mmHg risk of inadequate perfusion*
- Hyperosmotic agents
  — 20% mannitol
- Steroids
  — Dexamethosone (Decadron)
  — Methylprednisolone (Solu-Medrol)
- Barbiturates *— sedation*
- Prophylactic Phenytoin sodium (Dilantin) *– prevent seizures*
- Diuretics
  — Alternate with mannitol
  — Avoid narcotics! *—Alter CNS assessment*
- Controlled hyperventilation
- Mild hypothermia
- CSF drainage
  –risk of meningitis

Which change in the status of a client being treated for increased ICP warrants immediate action by the nurse?
A. Urinary output changes from 20 to 50 mL/hr
B. Arterial P_{CO_2} changes from 40 to 30 mmHg
C. Glasgow Coma Scale score changes from 5 to 7
D. Pulse changes from 88 to 68 beats/min

component of Cushing's triad; may indicate inc ICP

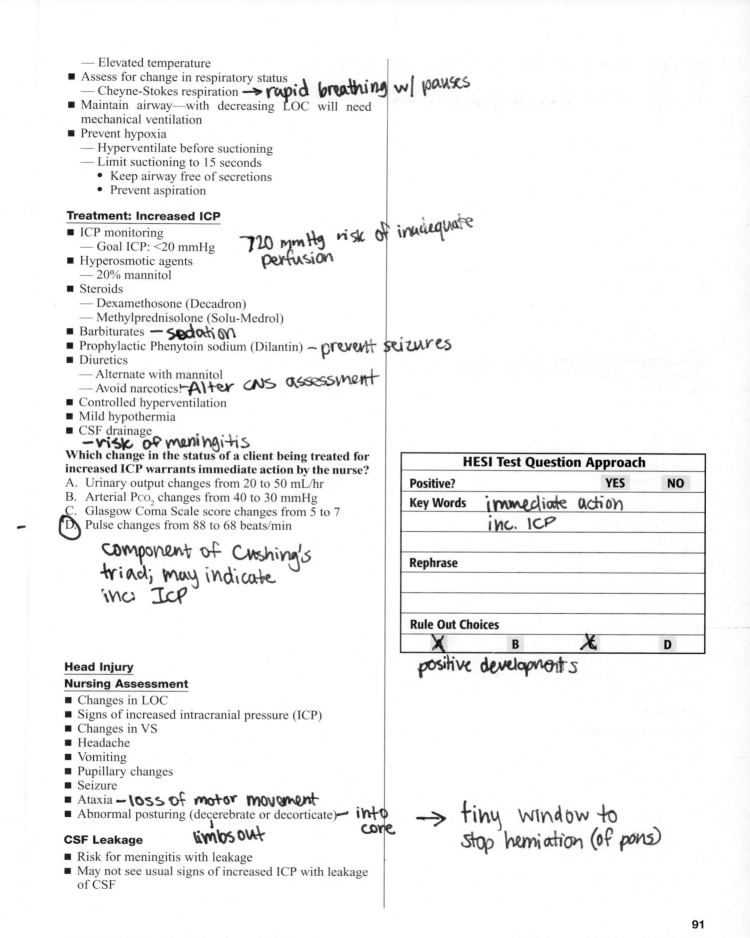

HESI Test Question Approach			
Positive?		YES	NO
Key Words	*immediate action inc. ICP*		
Rephrase			
Rule Out Choices			
A̶	B	C̶	D

positive developments

Head Injury
Nursing Assessment

- Changes in LOC
- Signs of increased intracranial pressure (ICP)
- Changes in VS
- Headache
- Vomiting
- Pupillary changes
- Seizure
- Ataxia *—loss of motor movement*
- Abnormal posturing (decerebrate or decorticate) *— into core*   → *tiny window to stop herniation (of pons)*
  limbs out

CSF Leakage

- Risk for meningitis with leakage
- May not see usual signs of increased ICP with leakage of CSF

91

- Drainage may come from nose (rhinorrhea) or ears (otorrhea)
- Altered cerebral perfusion related to ↑ ICP
  — MAP − ICP = CPP **(cerebral perfusion pressure)**
  — Amount of blood flow from systemic circulation required to provide oxygen to the brain
  — Ideally CPP should be > 70 mmHg

Nursing Interventions
- Neurological assessment every 15 minutes
- Notify healthcare provider at *first* sign of deterioration
- Limit visitors
- Keep room quiet
- Prevent straining
- Keep HOB at 30 to 45 degrees
- Avoid neck flexion/straining
- Monitor I & O

The nurse is planning a class on stroke prevention for clients with hypertension. What information is most important to provide to the class?
A. Salt restriction diet
B. Weight reduction
C. Medication compliance
D. Risk for stroke

life-long compliance of medication required for htn.

HESI Test Question Approach			
Positive?		YES	NO
Key Words	*Stroke prevention hypertension*		
Rephrase			
Rule Out Choices			
A	B	C	D

Stroke (Brain Attack) or Cerebrovascular Accident
- **Stroke** is a sudden loss of brain function caused by a disruption in the blood supply to part of the brain. Strokes are classified as ischemic or hemorrhagic.
  — *Ischemic stroke:* A clot may be thromboembolic or embolic, causing minimal or absent blood flow to the neurons.
  — *Hemorrhagic stroke:* May be a subarachnoid hemorrhage (SAH) or bleeding into the subarachnoid space, or an intracranial hemorrhage or direct bleeding into the brain tissue.
- **Transient ischemic attack (TIA):** A transient episode of neurological dysfunction caused by focal brain, spinal cord, or retinal ischemia, but without acute infarction of the brain. Clinical symptoms typically last less than 1 hour.

Nursing Assessment
- Risk factors
  — CVD, hypertension, previous TIA
  — Diabetes
  — Advanced age
  — History of atrial fibrillation or flutter
  — Oral contraceptives and hormone replacement therapy
  — Smoking
  — Alcohol: >2 drinks/day

The presenting symptoms relate to the specific area of the brain that has been damaged.

- Motor loss—hemiparesis or hemiplegia
- Communication loss—dysarthria, dysphasia, aphasia, or apraxia
- Perceptual disturbance—visual, spatial, and sensory
- Impaired mental acuity or psychological loss—decreased attention span, memory loss, depression, lability, hostility
- Bladder dysfunction may be either incontinence or retention

Nursing and Collaborative Management

- IV tissue plasminogen activator (tPA) improves the neurological outcome in clients with stroke, who meet fibrinolytic criteria, when administered within 3 hours -4.5 hours of onset. The client must be screened for intracranial bleeding before administration.
- Rehabilitation starts as soon as the client is stable.
- Mobility
- Speech
- ADL
- Elimination

Which client should be assigned to a graduate nurse being oriented to the neurological unit?

A. A client with a head injury who has a Glasgow Coma Scale score of 6

B. A client who developed autonomic dysreflexia after a T6 spinal cord injury

C. A client with multiple sclerosis who needs the first dose of interferon

D. A client suspected of having Guillain-Barré syndrome

[handwritten:] administer & teach about med assess for adverse effects

[handwritten right margin:]
Right-brain damage:
paralyzed on left
left-sided neglect
tend to deny
short attention span
impaired judgment

Left Brain Damage:
paralyzed right side
impaired speech
aware of deficits

HESI Test Question Approach			
Positive?		**YES**	**NO**
Key Words			
Rephrase			
Rule Out Choices			
A	B	C	D

Parkinson's Disease

- Chronic, progressive, debilitating neurological disease
- Triad of symptoms
  — Rigidity
  — Masklike face
    • Akinesia
    • Difficulty initiating and continuing movement
    • Bradykinesia
  — Tremors
    • Resting tremors
    • Pill rolling

Nursing and Collaborative Management
- *Safety* is always a priority!
- Take medications with meals
- Change positions slowly to reduce postural hypotension
- Thicken liquids
- Soft foods
- Encourage activity and exercise

Drug Therapy
- **Dopaminergics**
  — Levodopa (L-dopa, dopamine)
  — Blocks breakdown of levodopa to allow more levodopa to cross the blood-brain barrier
  — Avoid foods high in vitamin B_6 and high-protein foods   → *avoid foods high in protein*
  — Levodopa-carbidopa (Sinemet, Parcopa [orally dissolving tablet])
  — Allows for less use of levodopa and helps decrease side effects
- **Dopaminergic Agonists**
  — Bromocriptine mesylate (Parlodel)
    - Helps with motor fluctuations
  — Pramipexole (Mirapex)
  — Ropinirole hydrochloride (Requip)
  — Amantadine (Symmetrel)
- **Anticholinergics**—treat tremors
  — Trihexyphenidyl (Trihexyphen [Canada]; Artane)
  — Benztropine mesylate (Cogentin)
  — Procyclidine Hydrochloride (Akineton)
- **Antihistamine** *(tremors)*
  — Diphenhydramine (Benadryl)
- **Monoamine oxidase inhibitors**   → *use sparingly*
  — Selegiline hydrochloride (Anipril [Canada]; Eldepryl)
- **Catechol-O-methyl transferase** (COMT) inhibitors
  — Entacapone (Comptan)

The nurse is caring for a client hospitalized with Guillain-Barré syndrome. Which information would be most important for the nurse to report to the primary healthcare provider?
A. Ascending numbness from the feet to the knees
B. A decrease in cognitive status
C. Blurred vision and sensation changes
D. A persistent unilateral headache

hypoxia or hypercarbia may be present.

HESI Test Question Approach		
Positive?	**YES**	**NO**
Key Words		
Rephrase		
Rule Out Choices		
A	B	C	D

Guillain-Barré Syndrome

Involves peripheral and cranial nerves
- Usually occurs after an upper respiratory infection
- Ascending paralysis
- Rapid demyelination of the nerves
- Paralysis of the respiratory system may occur quickly
- Prepare to intubate

Nursing and Collaborative Management
- Plasmapheresis over 10 to 15 days
- IV high-dose immunoglobulin (Sandoglobulin) is as effective as plasma exchange and has the advantage of immediate availability and greater safety. Clients receiving high-dose immunoglobulin need to be well hydrated and have adequate renal function.
- Maintain patent airway
- Reposition frequently
- Impaired swallowing may require TPN
- Supervise feedings

[handwritten note: well hydrated w/ adequate urine output]

Multiple Sclerosis
- Demyelination of the central nervous system (CNS) myelin
- Disease is characterized by periods of remissions and exacerbations
- Assessment findings
  — Changes in visual field
  — Weaknesses in extremities
  — Numbness
  — Visual or swallowing difficulties
  — Unusual fatigue
  — Gait disturbances

Nursing and Collaborative Management
- Encourage self-care and frequent rest periods
- Take precautions against falls
- Voiding schedule; as incontinence worsens, teach clean self-catheterization
- Refer client for home healthcare services and support services
- Administer steroid therapy and chemotherapeutic drugs in acute exacerbations to shorten attack

Pharmacological Therapy

Focuses on controlling symptoms
- **Corticosteroids**
  — ACTH, prednisone, methylprednisolone
- **Immunomodulators**
  — Interferon-beta (Betaseron, Avonex, Rebif)
  — Glatiramer acetate (Copaxone)
- **Immunosuppressants**
  — Mitoxantrone hydrochloride
- **Cholinergics**
  — Bethanechol chloride (Duvoid [Canada]; Urecholine)
  — Neostigmine
- **Anticholinergics**
  — Propantheline
  — Oxybutynin chloride (Ditropan)

- **Muscle relaxants**
  — Diazepam (Valium)
  — Baclofen (Lioresal)
  — Dantrolene sodium (Dantrium)
  — Tizanidine (Zanaflex)
- **CNS stimulants**
  — Methylphenidate hydrochloride (Ritalin)
  — Modafinil (Alertec)
- **Antiviral/antiparkinsonian drugs**
  — Amantadine (Symmetrel); focus on prevention of infection

Myasthenia Gravis
- A chronic neuromuscular autoimmune disease
- Caused by loss of ACH receptors in the postsynaptic neurons at the neuromuscular junction
- ACH is necessary for muscles to contract
- Causes weakness and abnormal fatigue of voluntary muscles

Caused by excess cholinesterase

Nursing Assessment
- Ocular muscle weakness
- Bulbar muscle weakness *(cough & gag) → inability to maintain airway*
- Skeletal muscle weakness

Diagnosis
- Based on clinical presentation
  — Muscle weakness
- Confirmed by testing response to anticholinesterase drugs
- Tensilon test—2 mg IV

Nursing and Collaborative Management
Medications
- **Anticholinesterase agents**
  — Try to achieve maximum strength and endurance
  — Blocks action of cholinesterase
  — Increase levels of ACH at junctions
  — Common medications
    • Pyridostigmine bromide (Mestinon)
      □ Start with minimal doses
      □ Onset 30 minutes
      □ Duration 3 to 4 hours
      □ Must take on time!
- **Corticosteroid**
  — Prednisone
- **Immunosuppressive agents**
  — Azathioprine sodium (Imuran)
  — Cyclophosphamide (Procytox)

Types of Crisis
- Myasthenic
  — **Medical emergency**
  — Caused by undermedication or infection
  — Positive Tensilon test
  — Changes in VS, cyanosis, loss of cough and gag reflex, incontinence
  — May require intubation

AIRWAY!

- Cholinergic
  - Results from overmedication
  - Toxic levels of anticholinesterase medications
  - Symptoms: abdominal cramps, diarrhea, excessive pulmonary secretions
  - Negative Tensilon test

Atropine sulfate is reversal agent.

Nursing Interventions
- Coughing and deep breathing exercises
- Suction equipment at bedside
- Sit upright when eating and for 1 hour afterward
- Keep chin downward when swallowing
- Plan activities carefully; weakness is greater at the end of the day

Spinal Cord Injury
- Injuries classified by:
  - Extent of injury
  - Level of injury
  - Mechanism of injury
- Injuries classified as complete or incomplete
  - Transection/partial transection
- Rule of thumb
  - Injury above C8 = Quadriplegia
  - Injury below C8 = Paraplegia

Nursing Assessment
- Start with the ABCs
- Determine quality of respiratory status
- Check neurological status
- Assess vital signs
- Hypotension and bradycardia occur in injuries above T6

Nursing and Collaborative Management
- Immobilize and stabilize!
- Keep neck and body in anatomical alignment
- Maintain patent airway
- Cervical injuries are placed in skeletal traction
- High-dose corticosteroids are used to control edema during first 24 hours
- Spinal shock — *nervous system loses ability to transmit signals*
- Flaccid paralysis
  - Complete loss of reflexes
  - Hypotension
  - Bradycardia
  - Bowel and bladder distention
- Reverse as quickly as possible

Autonomic Dysreflexia
- Medical emergency that occurs in clients with injuries at or above T6
- Exaggerated autonomic reflex response
- Usually triggered by bowel or bladder distention
- S/S: Severe headache, ↑ BP, bradycardia, and profuse sweating
- Elevate head of bed (while maintaining correct alignment), relieve bowel or bladder distention

Monitor for UTI, urisepsis

Chapter **8** **Movement, Coordination, and Sensory Input**

Rehabilitation
- Watch for paralytic ileus
  - Assess bowel sounds
- Kinetic bed to promote blood flow
- Antiembolic stockings
- Protect from skin breakdown
- Bowel and bladder training
  - Keeping bladder empty and urine dilute and acidic to help prevent urinary tract infection, a common cause of death after spinal cord injury

Which action by the unlicensed assistive personnel (UAP) requires immediate follow-up by the nurse?
A. Positioning a client who is 12 hours postoperative from an above-the-knee amputation (AKA) with the residual limb elevated on a pillow
B. Assisting a client with ambulation while the client uses a cane on the unaffected side
C. Accompanying a client who has lupus erythematosus to sit outside in the sun during a break
D. Helping a client with rheumatoid arthritis to the bathroom after the client receives Celecoxib (Celebrex)

Sunlight may trigger lupus!

HESI Test Question Approach			
Positive?		YES	NO
Key Words	Immediate follow-up		
Rephrase			
Rule Out Choices			
A	B	C	D

Fractures
- Signs and symptoms
  - Pain, swelling, deformity of the extremity
  - Discoloration, loss of functional ability
  - Fracture evident on radiograph

Nursing Plans and Interventions
- Instruct in proper use of assistive devices
- Assess 5Ps of neurovascular functioning
  - Pain, paresthesia, pulse, pallor, paralysis
- Assess neurovascular area distal to injury
- Skin color, temperature, sensation, capillary refill, mobility, pain, and pulses
- Intervention
  - Closed reduction
  - Open reduction

Risk of Compartment Syndrome

- Postreduction
  - Cast
  - Traction
  - External fixation
  - Splints
  - Orthoses (braces)

Joint Replacement
- After surgery
  - Check circulation, sensation, and movement of extremity distal to replacement area
  - Assess 5 P's
  - Keep body in proper alignment
  - Encourage fluid intake
  - Use of bed pan, commode chair
  - Coordinate rehabilitation process

5Ps:
Pain
Pallor
Pulse
Paresthesia
Paralysis

hip replacement: aVoid raising leg and elevating knee

- Discharge home
  - Safety
  - Accessibility
- Drugs
  - Anticoagulants *—risk of thromboembolism*
  - Analgesics *—pain management*
  - Parenteral antibiotics *— prophylaxis*
- *Rehab*

Amputation

- Postoperative care
  - Monitor surgical dressing for drainage
  - Proper body alignment
  - Elevate residual limb (stump) first 24 hours
  - Do not elevate after 48 hours *(prevent contractures)*
  - Provide passive range of motion (ROM) and encourage prone position periodically to reduce risk of contracture
  - Ensure proper stump bandaging to prepare for prosthesis *; do not replace; reinforce*
  - Coordinate care with OT and PT
- Drug therapy
  - Analgesics
    - Phantom pain is real
  - Antibiotics

The nurse is assessing a client who is scheduled for surgical fixation of a compound fracture of the right ulna. Which finding should the nurse report to the healthcare provider?

A. Ecchymosis around the fracture site
B. Crepitus at the fracture site
C. Paresthesia distal to the fracture site *(circled)*
D. Diminished range of motion of the right arm

one of the 5Ps
diminished nerve function
compartment syndrome

HESI Test Question Approach			
Positive?		YES	NO
Key Words			
Rephrase			
Rule Out Choices			
A	B	C	D

A postmenopausal woman with a BMI of 18 has come to the clinic for her annual well woman examination. Which teaching plan topic should the nurse prepare for this high-risk client?

A. Osteoporosis *(circled)*
B. Obesity
C. Anorexia
D. Breast cancer

due to postmenopausal status.

HESI Test Question Approach			
Positive?		YES	NO
Key Words			
Rephrase			
Rule Out Choices			
A	B	C	D

Chapter **8** Movement, Coordination, and Sensory Input

Osteoporosis

Risk Factors

- Small, postmenopausal females
- Diet low in calcium
- Excessive alcohol, tobacco, and caffeine
- Inactive lifestyle
- Low testosterone level (men)

Nursing Assessment

- Dowager's hump
- Kyphosis of the dorsal spine
- Loss of height
- Pathological fractures
- Compression fracture of the spine can occur

Nursing Plans and Interventions

- Keep bed in low position
- Provide adequate lighting
- Avoid using throw rugs
- Provide assistance with ambulation
- Follow regular exercise program
- Diet high in vitamin D, protein, and calcium

Osteoporosis Drug Therapy

- **Bisphosphonates** Require client take with only water on arising in the morning, maintaining upright in the fasting state for 30-60 min (120 min for tiludronate)
  — Alendronate sodium (Fosamax)
  — Etidronate disodium (Didronel)
  — Zoledronic Acid (Aclasta, Zometa)
  — Ibandronate (Boniva)
  — Risedronate with calcium (Actonel Plus Calcium)
- **Selective estrogen receptor modulators** which have risk for thromboembolic events
  — Raloxifene hydrochloride (Evista)
- **Recombinant Parathyroid Hormone** Transient hypercalcemia, joint pain are common side effects
  — Teriparatide (Forteo)

The nurse is conducting an osteoporosis screening clinic at a health fair. What information should the nurse provide to individuals who are at risk for osteoporosis? (Select all that apply).

A. Limit alcohol and stop smoking
B. Suggest supplementing the diet with vitamin E
C. Promote regular weight-bearing exercise
D. Implement a home safety plan to prevent falls
E. Propose a regular sleep pattern of 8 hours nightly

HESI Test Question Approach		
Positive?	YES	NO
Key Words		
Rephrase		
Rule Out Choices		
A	B	C	D

Rheumatoid Arthritis

- Chronic, systemic, progressive deterioration of the connective tissue
- Etiology: unknown; believed to be autoimmune

Nursing Assessment

- Young to middle age
- More females than males
- Systemic with exacerbations and remissions
- Small joints first, then spreads
- Stiffness (may decrease with use)
- Decreased range of motion
- Joint pain
- Elevated erythrocyte sedimentation rate (ESR)
- Positive rheumatoid factor (RF) in 80% of clients
- Narrowed joint space

Nursing and Collaborative Management
Drug Therapy

- **High-dose ASA or NSAIDs**
- **Systemic corticosteroids**
- **Disease-modifying antirheumatic drugs (DMARDs)** → helps to keep pts. in remission
  - Methotrexate (Rheumatrex)
  - Sulfasalazine (Salazopyrin [Canada]; Azulfidine)
  - Hydroxychloroquine (Plaquenil)
  - Leflunomide (Arava)

Additional Interventions

- Heat and cold applications
- Weight management
- Rest and joint protection
- Use assistive devices
- Shower chair
- Canes, walkers
- Straight back chairs, elevated seats

Lupus Erythematosus

- Two classifications
  - *Discoid lupus erythematosus (DLE):* Affects skin only
  - *Systemic lupus erythematosus (SLE):* More prevalent than DLE
- Major trigger factors
  - Sunlight
  - Infectious agents
  - Stress
  - Drugs
  - Pregnancy

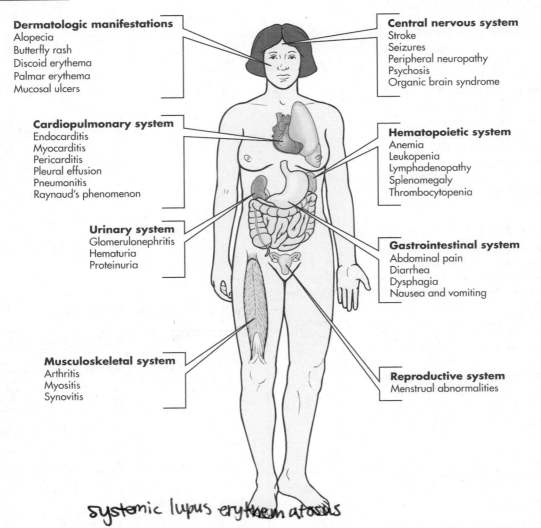

Dermatologic manifestations
Alopecia
Butterfly rash
Discoid erythema
Palmar erythema
Mucosal ulcers

Central nervous system
Stroke
Seizures
Peripheral neuropathy
Psychosis
Organic brain syndrome

Cardiopulmonary system
Endocarditis
Myocarditis
Pericarditis
Pleural effusion
Pneumonitis
Raynaud's phenomenon

Hematopoietic system
Anemia
Leukopenia
Lymphadenopathy
Splenomegaly
Thrombocytopenia

Urinary system
Glomerulonephritis
Hematuria
Proteinuria

Gastrointestinal system
Abdominal pain
Diarrhea
Dysphagia
Nausea and vomiting

Musculoskeletal system
Arthritis
Myositis
Synovitis

Reproductive system
Menstrual abnormalities

systemic lupus erythematosus

Figure 8-1 Common assessment findings in SLE. (From Lewis S, Dirksen S, Heitkemper M, et al: *Medical-surgical nursing: Assessment and management of clinical problems,* ed 8, St Louis, 2011, Mosby.)

- DLE: Scaly rash, butterfly rash over bridge of nose
- SLE: Joint pain, fever, nephritis, pericarditis
- Photosensitivity

Nursing and Collaborative Management

- Teaching
  — Drugs
  — Pain management
  — Disease process
  — Conserve energy
  — Avoid exposure to ultraviolet rays
  — Avoid/reduce stress
  — Use mild soaps, creams for skin care
  — Use of steroids for joint inflammation

- Therapeutic exercise and heat therapy
- Marital and pregnancy counseling

Kidney involvement is the leading cause of death in clients with lupus; the second leading cause is cardiac involvement.

Degenerative Joint Disease (Osteoarthritis)
- Joint pain—increases with activity
- Morning stiffness
- Crepitus
- Limited movement
- Joint enlargement

Caused by repetitive movement over time

Nursing and Collaborative Management
- Weight reduction diet
- Excessive use of involved joint may accelerate degeneration
- Use proper body mechanics
- Keep joints in functional position
- Hot and cold applications for pain and stiffness
- NSAIDs, opioid analgesics, and intraarticular corticosteroids

joint replacement needed

The nurse observes an elderly male client with glaucoma administer eye drops by tilting his head back, instilling each drop close to the inner canthus, and keeping his eye closed for 15 seconds. What action should the nurse take first?

A. Ask the client whether another family member is available to administer the drops
B. Review the correct steps of the procedure with the client
C. Administer the eye drops correctly in the other eye to demonstrate the technique
D. Discuss the importance of correct eye drop administration for persons with glaucoma

shouldn't instill in inner canthus

immediate feedback & re-teaching

HESI Test Question Approach		
Positive?	**YES**	**NO**
Key Words		
Rephrase		
Rule Out Choices		
A	B	C	D

Glaucoma
- Primary open-angle glaucoma
  — Drainage channels become clogged
  — Aqueous humor flow is reduced in trabecular meshwork
- Primary closure-angle glaucoma
  — Bulging lens from age related processes disrupts flow
- Silent thief of vision
- Normally painless
- Loss of peripheral vision
- May see halos around lights
- Diagnosed with eye examination
  — Tonometer to measure intraocular pressure

Nursing and Collaborative Management

- Keys to treatment
  - ↓ Intraocular pressure
  - ↓ Aqueous humor production
  - ↑ Drainage of aqueous humor
  - Teach client and family proper eye drop instillation
  - Teach client to avoid activities that can increase intraocular pressure
- Ambulatory/home care for open-angle glaucoma
  - Drug therapy
    - β-Adrenergic blockers
    - α-Adrenergic agonists
    - Cholinergic agents (miotics)
    - Carbonic anhydrase inhibitors
  - Surgical therapy
  - Argon laser trabeculoplasty (ALT)
  - Trabeculectomy with or without filtering implant
- Acute care for closure-angle glaucoma
  - Topical cholinergic agent
  - Hyperosmotic agent
  - Laser peripheral iridotomy
  - Surgical iridectomy

Glaucoma Drug Therapy

- **β-Adrenergic blockers**
  - Betaxolol hydrochloride (Betoptic)
  - Timolol maleate (Apo-Timop [Canada]; Timoptic, Istalol)
- **α-Adrenergic agonists**
  - Dipivefrin hydrochloride (Propine)
  - Epinephryl (Epinal)
- **Cholinergic agents (miotics)**
  - Carbachol (Miostat)
  - Pilocarpine hydrochloride (Akarpine, Diocarpine, Minims [Canada]; Isopto Carpine, Pilocar)
- **Carbonic anhydrase inhibitors**
  - Systemic
    - Acetazolamide (Acetazolam [Canada]; Diamox)
    - Methazolamide
  - Topical
    - Brinzolamide (Azopt)
    - Dorzolamide (Trusopt)
- **Combination therapy**
  - Timolol maleate and dorzolamide (Cosopt)
- **Hyperosmolar agents**
  - Glycerin liquid
  - Mannitol solution (Osmitrol)

Cataracts

- Clouding or opacity of the lens
- Early signs
  - Blurred vision
  - Decreased color perception

- Late signs
  — Double vision
  — Clouded pupil

Nursing and Collaborative Management: Cataract Removal

- Preoperative
  — Assess medications being taken
  — Anticoagulants should be stopped before surgery
  — Teach how to instill eye drops
- Postoperative
  — Eye shield should be worn during sleeping hours
  — Avoid lifting >10 lb
  — Avoid lying on operative side
  — Report signs of increased intraocular pressure
  — Acute pain

The nurse is teaching an 86-year-old client who has glaucoma and bilateral hearing loss. Which intervention should the nurse implement?
A. Maintain constant eye contact
B. Stand on the side unaffected by glaucoma
C. Speak in a lower tone of voice
D. Keep the environment dimly lit

elderly pt. able to hear low pitched more easily.

HESI Test Question Approach			
Positive?		YES	NO
Key Words			
Rephrase			
Rule Out Choices			
A	B	C	D

Eye Trauma/Injury

- Trauma
  — Determine type of injury
  — Position client in sitting position to decrease intraocular pressure
  — Never attempt to remove embedded object
  — Irrigate eye if a chemical injury has occurred
- Detached retina
  — Described as curtain falling over visual field
  — Painless
  — May have black spots or floaters (indicates bleeding has occurred with detachment)
  — Surgical repair of retina
  — Keep eye patch over affected area

Hearing Loss

- Conductive hearing loss
  — Sounds do not travel to the inner ear
  — May benefit from hearing aid

- Sensorineural hearing loss
  - — Sound distorted from defect in inner ear
- Common causes
  - — Infections
  - — Ototoxic drugs
    - Gentamicin
    - Vancomycin
    - Lasix
  - — Trauma
  - — Aging process
- Assessment
  - — Inability to hear whisper from 1 to 2 feet
  - — Shouting in conversations
  - — Turning head to favor one ear
  - — Loud volume on TV

Rhinne — next to ear

Weber — forehead

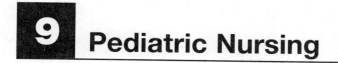

The nurse directs the unlicensed assistive personnel (UAP) to play with a 4-year-old child on bed rest. Which activity should the nurse recommend? (Select all that apply.)
A. Monopoly board game
B. Looking at picture books
C. Fifty-piece puzzle
D. Hand puppets *"make believe"*
E. Coloring book

HESI Test Question Approach			
Positive?		**YES**	**NO**
Key Words			
Rephrase			
Rule Out Choices			
A	**B**	**C**	**D**

Growth and Development
- **Five major developmental periods**
  - Prenatal
  - Infancy
  - Early childhood
  - Middle childhood
  - Later childhood (pubescence and adolescence)
- **Developmental theories most widely used to explain child's growth and development**
  - Freud's psychosexual stages
  - Erikson's stages of psychosocial development
  - Piaget's stages of cognitive development
  - Kohlberg's stages of moral development

Normal Growth and Development
Know norms for growth and development
- **Infant (birth to 1 year)**
  - Birth weight doubles by 6 months, triples by 12 months
  - Social smile occurs at 2 months
  - Plays "peek-a-boo" by 6 months
  - Sits upright without support by 8 months
  - Develops stranger anxiety at 7 to 9 months
  - Fine pincer grasp by 10 to 12 months (can pick up Cheerios)
  - Crawls at 10 months
  - Says a few words in addition to "mama" or "dada" at 12 months
- **Toddler (1-3 years)**
  - Throws ball overhand at 18 months
  - Two- to three-word sentences at 2 years
  - Toilet training starts around 2 years
  - Toddlers are ritualistic
  - No concept of time
  - Frequent tantrums

- **Preschool-age child (3-5 years)**
  - — Rides tricycle at 3 years
  - — Favorite word: *Why?*
  - — Sentences of five to eight words
- **School-age child (6-12 years)**
  - — Each year gains 4 to 6 lb, grows 2 inches
  - — Learns to tell time
  - — Socialization with peers very important
- **Adolescent (12-19 years)**
  - — Rapid growth, second only to the first year of life
  - — Secondary sex characteristics develop

[handwritten, right margin] → begin to develop moral conscience Sometimes development of sexuality

[handwritten, right margin] → psychosocial, spiritual development

A 7-year-old is to have a <u>painful</u> procedure. Which statement by the nurse best prepares the child to cope with this?
A. "It feels like burning pain."
B. "Sometimes this feels like pushing."
C. "There is nothing wrong when you have pain."
D. "You will get ice cream after the procedure."

[handwritten] avoid pain in description
don't bribe
↓
use non-pain descriptors

HESI Test Question Approach		
Positive?	YES	NO
Key Words		
Rephrase		
Rule Out Choices		
A	B	C	D

Pain Assessment and Management
- Assessment is based on verbal and nonverbal cues from child and parents' information
- Be aware of developmental responses to pain (i.e., intense, sustained crying in infants)
- Use appropriate pain scale
- Safety is the priority in administering medication
- Make sure dose is safe for age and weight

Nursing Interventions
Nonpharmacological Interventions
- Infants may respond best to pacifiers, holding, and rocking
- Toddlers and preschoolers may respond best to distraction
- School-age children and adolescents may use guided imagery

Pharmacological Interventions
- Before administering a pain medication to a pediatric client, verify that the prescribed dose is safe for the child on the basis of the child's weight.
- Monitor the child's vital signs after administration of opioid medications.
- Children as young as 5 years of age may be taught to use a client-controlled analgesia (PCA) pump.

[handwritten, right margin] → allows child to have more control of their pain

Immunization Teaching

- To prepare for NCLEX-RN exam, use knowledge from the immunization chart: *http://www.cdc.gov/vaccines/schedules/index.html*
  - *Example:* What vaccines would the nurse expect to be prescribed for a 2-month-old brought into the pediatrician's office for a well-baby checkup?
    Answer: DTaP, HepB, HIB, IPV, and PCV
  - *Example:* Withhold MMR vaccine for a person with a history of an anaphylactic reaction to neomycin or eggs.
- Common cold does *not* contraindicate immunization unless the fever is > 37.2° C (99° F)
- A fever < 38.9° C (< 102° F) and redness and soreness at the injection site are normal for 2 to 3 days after vaccination
- Call healthcare provider if child has high-pitched crying, seizures, or high fever → *likely caused by DTaP (Pertussis)*
- Use acetaminophen orally

Herd Immunity
- If 80% of population are immunized, others are protected

Communicable Diseases

- The incidence of common childhood communicable diseases has declined greatly since the advent of immunizations, but they do occur, and nurses should be able to identify the infection.
  - Measles
  - Rubeola
  - Rubella
  - Roseola
  - Mumps
  - Pertussis
  - Chickenpox
  - Diphtheria
  - Erythema infectiosum (fifth disease)
- Treat fever from infection with acetaminophen *not* ASA (acetylsalicylic acid, aspirin).
- Isolation is required during the infectious phase of the disease.
- Teaching is the primary intervention for prevention of spread.
- Provide supportive measures while disease runs its course.

Poisonings

- Frequent cause of childhood injury—teach poison-proofing methods for the home
- GI disturbance is a common symptom
- Burns of the mouth and pharynx with caustic poisonings
- Identify poisonous agent quickly.
- Check ABCs
- Teach parents not to make child vomit, because this may cause more damage
- Call Poison Control Center or 911, depending on how the child is acting

The nurse is performing the initial assessment of a 2-year-old child with suspected bacterial epiglottitis. Which technique is needed?

A. Use a tongue depressor to assess for erythema *Nothing in mouth—could cause airway ~~suffocation~~ obstruction*
B. Obtain a throat swab for culture and sensitivity
C. Observe for the presence of drooling
D. Measure pain using a FACES scale *(used for 3yrs & over)*

→ clinical indicators: drooling, dysphagia, distress

HIB vaccine prevents epiglottitis

HESI Test Question Approach			
Positive?		**YES**	**NO**
Key Words			
Rephrase			
Rule Out Choices			
A	B	C	D

Respiratory Dysfunction

- Infection of the respiratory tract
- Croup syndromes
- Tuberculosis
- Asthma
- Cystic fibrosis

A 4-year-old is brought to the clinic with a fever of 39.4° C (103° F), sore throat, and moderate respiratory distress caused by a suspected bacterial infection. Which medical diagnosis is a contraindication to obtaining a throat culture in the child?

A. Tonsillitis
B. Streptococcal infection
C. Bronchiolitis
D. Epiglottitis

— ≠ See above

HESI Test Question Approach			
Positive?		**YES**	**NO**
Key Words			
Rephrase			
Rule Out Choices			
A	B	C	D

Respiratory Disorders

- Be familiar with normal values for respiratory and pulse rates for children.
- Cardinal signs of respiratory distress
  — Restlessness
  — Increased respiratory rate
  — Increased pulse rate
  — Diaphoresis
- Respiratory failure usually occurs before cardiac failure.

Respiratory Infections

- Nasopharyngitis
- Tonsillitis
  — May be viral or bacterial
  — Treatment is important if related to streptococcal infection
  — Surgical treatment
    • Check prothrombin time (PT) and partial thromboplastin time (PTT) before surgery
    • Monitor for bleeding *→ frequent swallowing*
    • Highest risk for bleeding is during first 24 hours and 5 to 10 days postoperative

clear; nothing red/blue

no straws; milk products cause frequent clearing throat)

- Otitis media
  — S/S: Fever, pulling at ear
  — Discharge from ear
  — Administer antibiotics
  — Reduce temperature to prevent seizures
- Bacterial tracheitis
- Bronchitis
- Respiratory syncytial virus bronchiolitis
  — Isolate child (contact isolation)
  — Monitor respiratory status
  — Antiviral agent (ribavirin aerosols)
  — Maintain patent airway
  — RSV prophylaxis with monoclonal antibody palivizumab (Synagis) in high-risk children < 2 years old *[handwritten: → usually given monthly (IM) during vulnerable months → vastus lateralis]*
- Epiglottitis
  — S/S: High fever, sore throat, muffled voice, tripod position
  — IV antibiotics
  — Do not examine throat; may cause complete airway obstruction
  — Be prepared for tracheostomy

Asthma

- Leading cause of chronic illness in children
- Allergies influence persistence and severity
- Complex disorder involving biochemical, immunological, infection, endocrine, and psychological factors

Nursing Assessment and Interventions

- S/S: Tight cough, expiratory wheezing, peak flow levels
- Monitor for respiratory distress, need for O_2 nebulizer therapy
- Evaluate effects of β-adrenergic agonists, such as albuterol, and salbutamol sulfate (Ventolin) and levalbuterol [Xopenex], as well as antiinflammatory corticosteroids

The nurse is teaching the school-age child and parent about the administration of inhaled beclomethasone dipropionate (QVAR) and ipratropium bromide albuterol for the treatment of asthma. Which statement by the parent indicates that teaching has been effective?

A. "I'll keep the inhalers in the refrigerator."
B. "My child only needs to use the inhalers when the peak flow numbers are in the red."
C. "My child will take the bronchodilator first, then the corticosteroid." *[handwritten: opens alveoli]*
D. "My child will take the corticosteroid first, wait a few minutes, and then take the bronchodilator.

HESI Test Question Approach			
Positive?		**YES**	**NO**
Key Words			
Rephrase			
Rule Out Choices			
A	B	C	D

Cystic Fibrosis (CF)

- Most frequently occurring inherited disease of Caucasian children
- Transmitted by an autosomal recessive gene
- Diagnosis of CF may be based on a number of criteria
  — Identification of CF mutations
  — Absence of pancreatic enzymes
  — Steatorrhea
  — Chronic pulmonary involvement
    - Prevent respiratory infections
- Positive newborn screening test
  — First sign may be meconium ileus at birth
  — High sweat chloride concentration (pilocarpine test or sweat test)
- Delayed growth—poor weight gain
- Pancreatic enzymes with each meal and snacks
- Fat-soluble vitamins
- Teach family percussion and postural drainage techniques

Cardiovascular Disorders

Congenital Heart Disorders

May be classified as acyanotic or cyanotic
- Acyanotic (all have L-to-R shunt; increased pulmonary blood flow)
  — Ventricular septal defect
  — Atrial septal defect
  — Patent ductus arteriosus
  — Coarctation of the aorta
  — Aortic stenosis
- Cyanotic
  — Tetralogy of Fallot
  — Truncus arteriosus
  — Transposition of the great vessels

For illustrations of cardiovascular disorders, see a textbook or an NCLEX review manual:
- *Evolve Reach Comprehensive Review for the NCLEX-RN Examination (powered by HESI)*
- *Mosby's Comprehensive Review of Nursing for the NCLEX-RN Examination*
- *Saunders Comprehensive Review for the NCLEX-RN Examination Nursing and Collaborative Management*

- Maintain nutritional status; feeding should not last > 30 min
- Plan frequent rest periods
- Administer digoxin, diuretics and angiotensin-converting enzyme (ACE) inhibitors as prescribed

Congestive Heart Failure

- Common complication of congenital heart disorders
- S/S: Pedal edema, neck vein distention, cyanosis, grunting
- Monitor vital signs, elevate head of bed, O_2
- Digoxin, diuretics, and ACE inhibitors
- Weigh daily on same scale

[Handwritten annotations:]

generalized cyanosis

(pulmonary stenosis, VSD, overriding aorta, right ventricle hypertrophy)

Acrocyanosis: blue hands & feet within normal limits

Tetralogy of Fallot: unoxygenated blood pumped into systemic circulation

Prevention of Respiratory Distress: thermoregulation

Patent Ductus Arteriosus
- allows oxygenated blood pumped into lungs
- leads to pulmonary hypertension

respiratory rate <60 bpm conserve energy
✶ for nipple feeding✶

Managing Digoxin Therapy in Children

- Count apical rate when child is at rest; withhold medication if pulse is < 90-110 beats/min in infants or < 70 beats/min in older children
  — Notify healthcare provider
- Do not skip or try to make up doses
- Give 1 to 2 hours before meals
- Watch for S/S of toxicity and teach them to parents
  — Vomiting, anorexia, diarrhea, muscle weakness, drowsiness *"floppy"*   *difficult to arouse*
- Provide adequate potassium in the diet

Rheumatic Fever

- Peaks in school-age children
- Most common cause of acquired heart disease
- Affects connective tissue
- S/S: Sore throat appears to be getting better, then fever develops along with rash, chorea, elevated erythrocyte sedimentation rate *→ valvular problem*

Testing for strep early on

Nursing and Collaborative Management

- Encourage compliance with drug regimens
  — Penicillin remains drug of choice; *other antibiotics*
  — Salicylates are used to control inflammatory process and to reduce fever and discomfort
  — Prednisone may be indicated in some clients with heart failure
- Facilitate recovery from illness
  — Bed rest or at least limited activity during acute illness
  — Provide emotional support, *friends are important*
  ~ *school work*

The nurse reviews the medication record of a 2-month-old and notes that the infant was given a scheduled dose of digoxin with a documented apical pulse of 76 beats/min. What action should the nurse take first?

A. Assess the current apical heart rate *→ verify current cardiac function*
B. Observe for the onset of diarrhea
C. Complete an adverse occurrence report
D. Determine the serum potassium level

Should be 120-160 bpm (normal HR)

HESI Test Question Approach		
Positive?	**YES**	**NO**
Key Words		
Rephrase		
Rule Out Choices		
A	B	C	D

A child with hydrocephalus is 1 day postoperative for revision of a ventriculoatrial shunt. Which finding is most important?

A. Increased blood pressure
B. Increased temperature
C. Increased serum glucose
D. Increased hematocrit

best indicator of shunt malfunction
vomiting w/o nausea a sign
of neuro deterioration

HESI Test Question Approach		
Positive?	YES	NO
Key Words		
Rephrase		
Rule Out Choices		
A	B	C	D

Neuromuscular Disorders

The nurse is caring for a 16-year-old client with Down syndrome who has a mental age of 5 in the acute care hospital. Which priority nursing action should be included in this client's plan of care?
A. Monitoring for hearing loss
B. Monitoring I & O
C. Providing a dependable routine
D. Providing small puzzles

HESI Test Question Approach		
Positive?	YES	NO
Key Words		
Rephrase		
Rule Out Choices		
A	B	C	D

Down Syndrome
- Flat, broad nasal bridge; upward, outward slanting eyes
- Commonly associated problems
  - Cardiac defects
  - Delayed development
  - Respiratory problems
- Feed to back and side of mouth due to tongue thrust
- Support child/parent relationship to achieve the highest level of functioning
- Always evaluate mental age
- Refer family to early intervention program

Trisomy 21

Ultrasound can suggest chromosomal abnormality

VSD 30-40% of children w/ Down Syndrome

→ spectrum for cognitive effects

Cerebral Palsy (CP)
- Diagnosis made on evaluation of child
  - Persistent neonatal reflexes after 6 months
  - Spasticity
  - Scissoring of legs
  - Tight abductor muscles of hips
  - Tightening of heel cord
  - No parachute reflex

Nursing Interventions

- Prevent aspiration with feedings
- Phenytoin (Dilantin) for seizures
- Diazepam (Valium) for muscle spasms
- Botulinum toxin A (Botox)

Spina Bifida Occulta

- No sac present
- Suspect if tuft of hair at base of spine

→ folic acid during pregnancy (prevents neural tube defects)

Meningocele

- Sac contains only meninges and spinal fluid
- No nerves in spinal sac

Myelomeningocele

- Sac contains spinal fluid, meninges, and nerves
- Client has sensory and motor defects
- Preoperative/postoperative care
  — Monitor urine output
  — Watch for ↑ ICP
  — Keep sac free of stool and urine
  — Measure head circumference every 8 hours and check fontanels

posterior fontanel sometimes closed at birth

Hydrocephalus

- Abnormal accumulation of cerebrospinal fluid (CSF)
- Symptoms
  — ↑ Intracranial pressure (ICP)
  — ↑ BP
  — ↓ Pulse
  — Changes in level of consciousness
  — Irritability and vomiting

Nursing and Collaborative Management

- Elevate head of bed
- Seizure precautions
- Prepare for shunt placement
  — Assess for shunt malfunctioning
  — Monitor for S/S of infection
- Teaching related to shunt replacement

Seizures/Epilepsy

- More common in children under 2 years
- Types of seizures
  — Generalized
    - Tonic/clonic (formerly grand mal)
    - Aura (tactile, optic, etc.)
    - Loss of consciousness
    - Tonic phase: stiffness of body
    - Clonic phase: spasms and relaxation
    - Postictal phase: sleepy and disoriented
  — Petit mal
    - Momentary loss of consciousness, appears like daydreaming, poor performance in school
    - Lasts 5 to 10 seconds
- Status epilepticus
- Series of seizures at intervals too brief to allow the child to regain consciousness

Nursing and Collaborative Management: Seizures

- Maintain patent airway
- Side rails up
- Pad side rails
- Administer anticonvulsants
- Teach family/client about medication

Anticonvulsants/Types of Seizures

- **Phenobarbital**
  — Generalized tonic clonic
  — Partial
  — Status epilepticus
- **Primidone** (Mysoline)
  — Generalized tonic clonic
  — Partial
  — Status epilepticus
- **Phenytoin** (Dilantin)
  — Generalized tonic clonic
  — Partial
  — Status epilepticus
- **Fosphenytoin** (Cerebyx) IM/IV
  — Generalized convulsive status epilepticus
  — Treatment of seizures during neurosurgery
  — Short-term parenteral replacement for phenytoin oral (Dilantin)
- **Valproic acid** (Depakene)
  — Generalized tonic clonic
  — Absence
  — Myoclonic
  — Partial
- **Clonazepam** (Rivotril [Canada]; Klonopin)
  — Absence
  — Myoclonic
  — Infantile spasms
  — Partial
- **Carbamazepine** (Tegretol)
  — Generalized tonic-clonic
  — Partial

Bacterial Meningitis

- Usually caused by *H. influenzae* type b, *Streptococcus pneumoniae,* and *Neisseria meningitidis* (See Table 9.1, Leading Causes of Pediatric Meningitis)
- Signs and symptoms
  — Petechial or purpuric rashes (meningococcal infection), especially when associated with shock like state
  — *Older children:* Include S/S of increased ICP, neck stiffness, + Kernig's sign, + Brudzinski's sign
  — *Infants:* Classic signs absent, poor feeding, vomiting, irritability, bulging fontanels
- Diagnostic procedures include lumbar puncture for laboratory analysis

nucal rigidity

First 24 hrs is critical
mortality high if not discovered early

Table 9.1 Leading Causes of Pediatric Meningitis

Age	Organism
Birth to 3 months	Enteric bacilli Group B streptococci
3 months to 10 years	Streptococcus pneumoniae, Neisseria meningitidis (meningococci)
10 years to 19 years	N. meningitidis, S. pneumoniae

Adapted from Hockenberry M, Wilson D: *Wong's Nursing Care of Infants and Children*, ed 9, St. Louis, 2011, Mosby.

Nursing and Collaborative Management

- Isolate at least 24 hours → *droplet (gown, gloves, mask)*
- Administer antibiotics
- Frequent VS and neurological checks
- Increased ICP, muscle twitching, and changes in LOC
- Measure head circumference daily
- Syndrome of inappropriate antidiuretic hormone (SIADH) occurs frequently
- Fluid restrictions may be necessary

Reye's Syndrome

- Etiology often, but not always, associated with aspirin use and influenza or varicella
- Rapidly progressing encephalopathy
- S/S: Lethargy progressing to coma, vomiting, hypoglycemia
- Neurological checks; maintain airway
- Mannitol for ICP control
- Early diagnosis is important to improve client outcome

HESI Test Question Approach			
Positive?		**YES**	**NO**
Key Words			
Rephrase			
Rule Out Choices			
A	B	C	D

Muscular Dystrophy (MD)

- Duchenne's MD
  - Onset between ages 2 and 6 years
  - Most severe and most common MD of childhood
  - X-linked recessive disorder *(female carrier; expressed in male children; 50% chance)*
- Diagnosis
  - Muscle biopsy: muscle fibers degenerate and are replaced by connective tissue and fat
  - Serum creatine phosphokinase (CK) levels are extremely high in the first 2 years of life before the onset

117

- ■ Symptoms
  - — Delayed walking
  - — Frequent falls
  - — Easily tires when walking
- ■ Interventions
  - — Exercise
  - — Prevent falls
  - — Assistive devices for ambulation

→ prone to accidents in wheelchair by adolescence

Renal Disorders in Children

Urinary Tract Infection (UTI)
- ■ More common in girls
- ■ Symptoms
  - — Poor food intake
  - — Strong-smelling urine
  - — Fever
  - — Pain with urination
- ■ Interventions
  - — Obtain urine culture before starting antibiotics *→ E.coli*
- ■ Teach home care
  - — Finish all antibiotics
  - — Avoid bubble baths
  - — Increase intake of acidic fluids, such as apple or cranberry juice

Vesicoureteral Reflux
- ■ Retrograde flow of urine into the ureters
- ■ Symptoms
  - — Recurrent UTIs
  - — Common with neurogenic bladder
- ■ Interventions
  - — Teach to prevent UTI
  - — Record output after catheterization
  - — Maintain hydration

bladder is not fully emptied
– dilated ureters

massage symphisis pubis
later on must learn self-cathenitzation

Acute Glomerulonephritis (AGN)
- ■ Common features
  - — Oliguria, hematuria, and proteinuria
  - — Edema
  - — Hypertension
  - — Circulatory congestion
  - — Therapeutic management
  - — Maintenance of fluid balance
  - — Treatment of hypertension
- ■ Assessment
  - — Recent strep infection
  - — Dark ("iced tea") urine *(indicates blood)*
  - — Irritable and/or lethargic

→ autoimmune response to strep

kidney not functioning properly

Nursing and Collaborative Management
- ■ VS every 4 hours
- ■ Daily weights
- ■ Low-sodium, low-potassium diet

Chapter **9** **Pediatric Nursing**

Nephrotic Syndrome

Characterized by increased glomerular permeability to protein
- Assessment
  - — Frothy urine
  - — Massive proteinuria
  - — Edema
  - — Anorexia

massive amounts of protein in urine

etiology unknown

may require dialysis

Nursing and Collaborative Management

- Reducing excretion of protein
- Reducing or preventing fluid retention
- Preventing infection
- Skin care
- Administer medications
  - — Diuretics
  - — Corticosteroid therapy
  - — Immunosuppressants
- Small frequent feeding

Discharge Teaching

- Daily weights
- Side effects of meds
- Prevent infections

Acute Renal Failure Management

- Treatment of the underlying cause
- Managing the complications of renal failure
- Providing supportive therapy

Abnormalities in Chronic Kidney Disease

- Waste product retention
- Water and sodium retention
- Hyperkalemia
- Acidosis
- Calcium and phosphorus disturbance
- Anemia
- Hypertension
- Growth disturbances

→ usually polycystic kidney disease transplant necessary

Home Dialysis

- Peritoneal dialysis is the preferred form of dialysis for infants, children and parents who wish to remain independent, or who live a long distance from a dialysis center, and children who prefer fewer dietary restrictions and a gentler form of dialysis.
- Hemodialysis is best suited to children who do not have someone in the family who is able to perform home peritoneal dialysis and to those who live close to a dialysis center. The disadvantages include school absence during dialysis and strict fluid and dietary restrictions between dialysis sessions.

Nursing and Collaborative Management

- Educate family
  - — Disease, its implications, therapeutic plan
  - — Possible psychological effects
  - — Treatment and technical aspects of the procedure

- Major concerns in kidney transplantation
  — Tissue matching
  — Prevention of rejection
- Psychological concerns
  — Self-image related to body changes caused by corticosteroid therapy

A school-age child with nephrotic syndrome is seen at the clinic 2 days after discharge from the hospital. Which assessment is most important to obtain after hemodialysis?
A. Pain assessment
B. Capillary refill
C. Urine ketones
D. Daily weight

determines effectiveness

HESI Test Question Approach		
Positive?	YES	NO
Key Words		
Rephrase		
Rule Out Choices		
A	B	C	D

Gastrointestinal Disorders

Nutritional Assessment
- Present nutritional status
- Body mass index
- Dietary history
- Past nutrition assessment
- Height
- Weight
- Head circumference
- Skinfold thickness
- Arm circumference *(after first year of life)* — *Iron in formula and breast milk → occurs @ change to whole milk*
- Iron deficiency
  — $FeSO_4$ drops: Use straw; give with orange juice, not with dairy foods

Diarrhea
- Worldwide leading cause of death in children <5 years of age
- Classified as acute or chronic
- Common problem for infants
- Assessment *depressed fontanel*
  — Depressed sunken eyes
  — Weight loss
  — Decreased urine output

6-8 wet diapers per day for infants

Nursing and Collaborative Management
- Fluid and electrolyte balance
- Rehydration
- Maintenance fluid therapy
- Reintroduction of adequate diet
- Do not give antidiarrheal agents

Cleft Lip or Cleft Palate
- Malformation of the face or oral cavity
- Initial closure of cleft lip is performed when infant weighs approximately 10 lb
- Closure of cleft palate at around 1 year
- Promote bonding
- Breck/Haberman feeder
- Maintain airway
- No straws, no spoons, only soft foods for cleft palate

can sometimes be seen on ultrasound

may use elbow restraint to prevent injury

Pyloric Stenosis
- Common in first-born males
- Vomiting becomes projectile around day 14 after birth

inconsolable crying

Perioperative Care of Client For Repair
Intussusception
- Telescoping of one part of intestine
- Emergency intervention is needed

more common in males

→ pass bloody stools
sausage-shaped mass in abdomen
→ barium enema given

Congenital Aganglionic Megacolon (Hirschsprung's Disease)
- Series of surgeries to correct
- Temporary colostomy

more common in males w/ Down Syndrome

→ failure to pass meconium; dead bowel

Hematological Disorders

→ temporary colostomy
→ occurs @ 12 wks gestation

Iron Deficiency Anemia
- Common in infants, toddlers, and adolescent females
- Review Hgb norms for children
- Teach family about administering oral iron

Sickle Cell Anemia
- Autosomal recessive disorder
- Fetal Hgb does not sickle
- Hydration to promote hemodilution
- Symptoms
  — Crisis marked by fever and pain
- Treatment during crisis
  — Bedrest to minimize energy expenditure
  — Improve oxygen utilization
  — Hydration through oral and IV therapy (priority)
  — Analgesia for severe pain from vasoocclusion
  — Blood replacement to treat anemia and to reduce the viscosity of the sickled blood
  — Antibiotic therapy to treat any existing infection
- Maintenance
  — Keep well hydrated
  — Do not give supplemental iron
  — Give folic acid orally

pregnancy a risk factor

hydration prevents sickling

Hemophilia
- X-linked recessive disorder
- Interventions
  — Administer fresh frozen plasma
  — Apply pressure to even minor bleeding
- Increased risk for bleeding

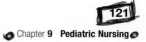

Metabolic and Endocrine Disorders

Phenylketonuria (PKU)

- Autosomal recessive disorder
- Newborn screening with Guthrie test
  — Performed at birth and at 3 weeks
- Strict adherence to low-phenylalanine diet
- Special PKU formula
- Avoid meat, milk, dairy, and eggs — can have breast-milk
- Use: fruits, juices, cereal, bread, and starches

relatively rare, except in Irish population
can lead to mental retardation if not addressed
vegan diet up to age 18

Diabetes
Obesity

- 19% of 6- to 11-year-olds categorized as overweight or obese
- Leads to adult obesity with increased risks of cardiovascular issues and type 2 diabetes
- Minorities disproportionally at risk
- Parental obesity is the highest predictor of childhood obesity
- BMI, dietary, and activity assessments should be obtained and evaluated

Type 2 diabetes: The defect is insulin resistance and relative insulin deficiency. There is insufficient insulin production, insulin resistance and/or excessive and unregulated glucose production from the liver.
- Risk of overweight: BMI-for-age 85th to 95th percentile
- Overweight: BMI-for-age > 95th percentile
- Acanthosis nigricans (a marker) is a risk factor for diabetes

Type 1 diabetes: Immune-mediated disease associated with absolute insulin deficiency. The body's own T cells destroy pancreatic beta cells, which are the source of insulin. Type 1 diabetes is common in school-age children. Classic symptoms are polyuria, polyphagia, polydipsia and weight loss. Child may wet the bed. Cognitive level and age should be considered when planning teaching.
- Dietary teaching
- Exercise management
- Insulin administration
- Continuous follow up important
- Monitoring
- Hypoglycemia

Skeletal Disorders

Nursing Assessment

- Visible signs of fractures
- Obtain baseline pulses, color, movement, sensation, temperature, swelling, and pain
- Report any changes immediately

Traction

- Buck's traction
  — For knee immobilization
- Russell's traction
  — For fracture of femur or lower leg
- Dunlap's traction
  — Can be skeletal or skin
- 90°/90° traction
- Provide appropriate toys, teach cast care to family, prevent cast soilage with diapering, monitor neurovascular status

Congenital Dislocated Hip

- Assessment
  — Positive Ortolani's sign
  — Unequal fold of skin on buttocks
  — Limited abduction of hip

Nursing and Collaborative Management

- Apply Pavlik harness (worn 24 hours a day)
- Surgical correction
- Postoperative intervention
- Hip spica cast care

Scoliosis

- **S**-shaped curvature of the spine
- Most common nontraumatic skeletal condition in children
- Affects both genders at all ages but is most commonly seen in adolescents

Juvenile Rheumatoid Arthritis (JRA)

- Most common arthritic condition of childhood
- Inflammatory diseases that involve the joints, connective tissues, and viscera
- Exact cause unknown, but infections and autoimmune response have been implicated
- Therapy consists of administration of medications (e.g., NSAIDs, methotrexate, or aspirin), along with exercise, heat application, and support of joints

[Handwritten notes:]

More common in females

sometimes cloth diapers used

Growth spurt:
6 months before, 6 after puberty
→ Milwaukee brace 23 hrs a day
→ can happen as young as 5-6 yrs old

The practical nurse (PN) is assigned to care for a 3-year-old with Reye's syndrome. The child's temperature is 39.1° C (102.4° F), and the PN is preparing to administer aspirin PO. What action should the charge nurse implement?

A. Direct the PN to assess the gag reflex and LOC
B. Advise the PN to wait until the fever is greater than 39.1° C (102.4° F)
C. Remind the PN to hold all aspirin-containing medication
D. Tell the PN to notify the healthcare provider

education about aspirin

HESI Test Question Approach			
Positive?		YES	NO
Key Words			
Rephrase			
Rule Out Choices			
A	B	C	D

While receiving IV antibiotics for sepsis, a 2-month-old is crying inconsolably despite the mother's presence. The nurse recognizes that the infant is exhibiting symptoms related to which condition?

A. Allergic reaction to the antibiotics
B. Pain related to IV infiltration
C. Separation anxiety from the mother
D. Hunger and thirst

Crying most likely signifies pain

HESI Test Question Approach			
Positive?		YES	NO
Key Words			
Rephrase			
Rule Out Choices			
A	B	C	D

rxn would occur sooner

mother is there

10 Maternal-Newborn Nursing

A client at 36 weeks' gestation is placed in the lithotomy position; she suddenly complains of feeling breathless and lightheaded and shows marked pallor. What action should the nurse take first?

A. Turn her to a lateral position *(either side)*
B. Place her in the Trendelenburg position
C. Obtain vital signs and a pulse oximetry reading
D. Initiate distraction techniques

supine hypotensive syndrome
- suppression of vena cava

HESI Test Question Approach			
Positive?		YES	NO
Key Words			
Rephrase			
Rule Out Choices			
A	B	C	D

Pregnancy: Key Assessments

- Assess for violence
  — Battering and emotional or physical abuse can begin with pregnancy
  — Assess for abuse in private, away from the partner, throughout pregnancy
  — Nurse needs to know:
    • Local resources
    • How to determine client's safety
- Gravidity and parity
  — *Gravida:* Number of times woman has been pregnant, regardless of outcome
  — *Para:* Number of deliveries (not children) occurring after 20 weeks of gestation
    • Multiple births count as one
    • Pregnancy loss before 20 weeks counted as abortion but add 1 to gravidity
    • Fetal demise after 20 weeks is added to parity
- GTPAL equals number of
  G Gravidity pregnancy
  T Term pregnancies *≥ 38 wks*
  P Preterm pregnancies *< 38 wks*
  A Abortions (elective or spontaneous)
  L Living children *↳ miscarriage*
- Gestation
  — Naegele's rule
    • Count back 3 months from date of last normal menstrual period
    • Add 1 year and 7 days
    Example: If the last menstrual period was May 2, 2013, EDB would be February 9, 2014.

- Fundal height
  - 12-13 weeks: Fundus rises out of symphysis
  - 20 weeks: Fundus at umbilicus
  - 24 to ~36 weeks: Fundal height (cm) measured from the symphysis equals the number of weeks of gestation (if a single pregnancy)
- Weight gain
  - Optimal weight gain is not known precisely
    - 1st trimester the average total weight gain is 1 to 2.5 kg
    - Approximately 0.4 kg per week for a woman of normal weight during 2nd and 3rd trimesters
- Psychological maternal changes
  - Ambivalence: Occurs early in pregnancy, even with a planned pregnancy.
  - Acceptance: Occurs with the woman's readiness for the experience and her identification with the motherhood role.
  - *Emotional lability:* Frequent changes of emotional states or extremes in emotional states.
- Common diagnostic tests
  - Alfa-Fetoprotein (AFP) test predicts neural tube defects with high incidence of false positive at 16-18 weeks
  - Chorionic villi sampling (CVS) determines sickle-cell, PKU, Down Syndrome, muscular dystrophy; at 8-12 weeks; full bladder required; Rh- mother requires RhoGAM post procedure
  - Amniocentesis performed at 16 weeks to determine genetic disorders, at 30 weeks to determine lung maturity; bladder emptied if performed after 20 weeks gestation; Rh- mother requires RhoGAM (WinRho, [Canada]) post procedure
  - Ultrasound – multiple purposes; must have full bladder
- Non-stress test via ultrasound transducer records fetal movement and heart rate after 28 weeks
- Contraction stress test evaluates fetal response to stress of labor

(handwritten note: Open-ended questions → takes better care of herself)

A client's suspected pregnancy is confirmed. The client tells the nurse that she also has had one pregnancy that she delivered at 39 weeks; twins that she delivered at 34 weeks; and a single gestation that she delivered at 35 weeks. Using the GTPAL notation, how should the nurse record the client's gravidity and parity?

A. 3-0-3-0-3
B. 3-1-1-1-3
C. 4-1-2-0-4
D. 4-2-1-0-3

HESI Test Question Approach			
Positive?		YES	NO
Key Words			
Rephrase			
Rule Out Choices			
A	B	C	D

The nurse is monitoring a client in the first stage of labor. The RN identifies fetal heart rate (FHR) decelerations at the onset of each contraction and a return to the baseline after the contraction. What action should the nurse take?

A. Discontinue the oxytocin infusion
B. Continue to monitor the FHR
C. Give a bolus of 750 mL D₅LR
D. Insert a fetal scalp electrode

head compression normal in birthing process

HESI Test Question Approach			
Positive?		**YES**	**NO**
Key Words			
Rephrase			
Rule Out Choices			
A	**B**	**C**	**D**

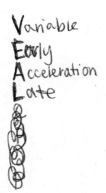

Variable
Early
Acceleration
Late

Cord compression
Head compression
Okay!
Placental insufficiency

Labor and Delivery

- Stages of Labor
  - *First Stage* - Stage of dilation and effacement and complete with 100% cervical effacement and complete dilation of cervix (10 cm). Duration is from 8 to 20 hours in the primipara and 5 to 14 hours in the multipara. (3 phases)
  - *Second Stage* –Stage of expulsion and ends with birth of the baby. Generally lasts from a few minutes to 2 hours.
  - *Third Stage* is labeled the placental separation stage. It begins with the birth of the baby and ends with the expulsion of the placenta. This process can last up to 30 minutes, with an average length of 5 to 10 minutes.
  - *Fourth Stage* arbitrarily lasts up to two hours after delivery of placenta. Monitor for excessive bleeding.

Labor Progression

- *Cervical dilation:* Stretching of the cervical os from fingertip diameter to large enough to allow passage of the infant (10 cm)
- *Effacement:* Thinning and shortening of the cervix (0% to 100%)
- *Station:* Location of the presenting part in relation to the midpelvis or ischial spines, measured in centimeters above and below
  - Station 0 = Engaged
  - Station +2 = 2 cm below the level of the ischial spines
- *Fetal presentation:* Part of the fetus that presents to the inlet
- *Position:* Relationship of the point of reference (occiput sacrum, acromion) on the fetal presenting part to the mother's pelvis
  - Left occiput anterior (LOA)—most common
- *Lie:* Relationship of the long axis (spine) of the fetus to the long axis (spine) of the mother
  - Longitudinal: Up and down
  - Transverse: Perpendicular
  - Oblique: Slanted
- *Attitude:* Relationship of fetal parts to one another
  - Flexion: Desired, so that smallest diameters are presented
  - Extension

Maternal-Fetal Monitoring

- Time contractions
  - *Frequency:* From the beginning of one contraction to the beginning of the next contraction
  - *Duration:* Amount of time a contraction lasts, from the beginning to the end
  - *Intensity:* Internal monitoring from 30 mmHg (mild) to 70 mmHg (strong)
  - *Resting tone/time:* Tension of uterine muscle between contractions and time between contractions
- Heart rate
  - Normal: 110-160 beats/min
  - Tachycardia: >160 beats/min
  - Bradycardia: <120 beats/min
- Nursing actions based on fetal heart rate; treat based on cause
  - Reassuring patterns
    - Accelerations
  - Nonreassuring patterns:
    - Late decelerations (nonreassuring, even if not very "deep") hypoxia
    - Early decelerations (may occur during second stage and indicate pushing)
    - Variable decelerations (occurring at any time and indicate an ominous pattern and indicate compression of umbilical cord

External fetal monitoring is noninvasive and is performed with a Toco transducer or Doppler ultrasonic transducer. *Internal fetal monitoring* is invasive and requires rupturing of the membranes and attachment of an electrode to the presenting part of the fetus.

A woman who is in labor becomes nauseated, starts hiccupping, and tells her partner to leave her alone. The partner asks the nurse what he did to make this happen. How should the nurse respond?

A. "In active labor, it is quite common for women to react this way. It's nothing you did."

B. "I don't know what you did, but stop, because she is quite sensitive right now."

C. "I'll come and examine her. This reaction is common during the transition phase of labor."

D. "Early labor can be very frustrating. I'm sure she doesn't mean to take it out on you."

[handwritten notes: introversion seriousness; excitement anxiety]

True Labor

- Pain in lower back radiating to abdomen
- Regular, rhythmic contractions
- Increased intensity with ambulation
- Progressive cervical dilation and effacement

False Labor

- Discomfort localized to abdomen
- No lower back pain
- Contractions decrease in intensity and/or frequency with ambulation

HESI Test Question Approach		
Positive?	YES	NO
Key Words		
Rephrase		
Rule Out Choices		
A	B	C	D

risk of cord prolapse —→ Trendelenberg position immediately —→ call for help

The nurse performs a vaginal examination for a laboring client. The RN determines that the cervix is dilated 4 cm with 60% effacement, and the presenting part is at the −2 station. Thirty minutes later, the client calls the RN and says, "I think my water just broke." Which action has the highest priority?

A. Call in the results to the healthcare provider
B. Evaluate the fetal heart rate
C. Help the client to the bathroom for hygiene
D. Perform the nitrazine and fern tests

↳ if water breaks at home or out of hospital (turns black in presence of amniotic fluid)

HESI Test Question Approach			
Positive?		YES	NO
Key Words			
Rephrase			
Rule Out Choices			
A	B	C̶	D

Management of Discomfort
Types of Regional Blocks
- Pudendal block
  - Given in second stage
  - Produce numbness of the genital and perianal region Has no effect on pain of uterine contractions
- Epidural Regional Anesthesia: Peridural (epidural or caudal) block
  - Given in first or second stage
  - Single dose or continuously
  - May prolong second stage
- Spinal Anesthesia (block): Intradural (subarachnoid, spinal)
  - Given in second stage
  - Rapid onset
  - Client remains flat for 6 to 8 hours after delivery

Administration of Analgesic Medication
Drugs Used During Labor
- **Fentanyl** (Duragesic) (Sublimaze)
- **Morphine sulphate** (MS Contin)
- **Butorphanol tartrate** (Apo-butorphanol [Canada]; Stadol)
- **Nalbuphine** (Nubain)
- **Dilaudid**

Postpartum Maternal Physical Assessment Summary
Fundal Involution
- Immediately: Fundus is several centimeters below umbilicus
- Within 12 hours: Fundus rises to umbilicus
- Descends 1 cm (fingerbreadth) a day for 9 to 10 days, then fundus is below symphysis pubis
- Should be in midline and firm.

Void before fundal assessment

Lochia
  - Endometrial sloughing from rubra to serosa to alba
  - Assess color, odor, volume
Breasts
  - Assess nipple soreness, fullness, engorgement, lumps *(prolactin for milk production; oxytocin for let down)*
Bladder
  - Measure output; assess for distention or retention *; full bladder may cause fundus to not be midline*
Bowel
  - Assess distention and bowel sounds

Episiotomy
— Assess episiotomy or laceration repair for intactness, hematoma, edema, bruising, redness, and drainage.

Bonding
— Assess attachment behaviors

Planning for Discharge
All health plans are required to allow the new mother and newborn to remain in the hospital for a minimum of 48 hours after a normal vaginal birth and for 96 hours after a cesarean birth unless the attending provider, in consultation with the mother, decides on early discharge

Teaching Points
- Change pads as needed and with voiding/defecation. Wipe front to back.
- Good hand-washing technique
- Ice packs, sitz baths, peri bottle lavage, and topical anesthetic spray and pads
- Breast-feeding instructions
- Balance diet and fluid intake
- Rest/nap when baby sleeps
- Contraceptive use
- Postpartum emotions: baby blues, postpartum depression
- Baby Care
  — Diapering, bathing, skin care, cord care
  — Circumcised or uncircumcised care
  — Burping, bowel movements, and wet diapers
  — Sleeping habits and newborn behavior
  — Jaundice

Rh-immune globulin WinRho (Canada); RhoGAM
- Given to Rh-negative women with possible exposure to Rh-positive blood
- Should have negative indirect Coombs test
- Given IM within 72 hours after delivery
- Checked by two nurses (blood product)

Rubella Vaccine
- Given subcutaneously to nonimmune client before discharge from hospital
- May breast-feed
- Do not give if client or family member is immuno-compromised
- Avoid pregnancy for 2 to 3 months (teach contra-ception)

A client who is 72 hours post cesarean section is preparing to go home. She shares that she cannot get the baby's diaper on "right." Which action should the nurse take?
A. Demonstrate how to diaper the baby correctly
B. Observe the client diapering the baby while offering praise and hints
C. Call the social worker for long-term follow-up
D. Reassure the client that she knows how to take care of her baby

[handwritten notes: "May need stool softener / Ice pack to decrease swelling" ; "May need more than once" ; "Taking hold" ; "(72 hrs PP)"]

HESI Test Question Approach		
Positive?	YES	NO
Key Words		
Rephrase		
Rule Out Choices		
A	B	C	D

Four births will occur at once. Which birth should the nursery charge nurse assign to a newly licensed nurse as her first solo birth and admission?

A. G1 P0 at 39 weeks who will give birth vaginally after a 15-hour <u>induced</u> labor. The mother has been on <u>magnesium sulfate</u> for <u>pre-eclampsia</u> throughout labor.

B. G5 P4 at 38 weeks who will give birth vaginally after a 5-hour unmedicated labor. Mild to moderate variable decelerations have been occurring for the past 15 minutes.

C. G3 P1 at <u>34 weeks</u> who will give birth by <u>cesarean section</u> for a <u>nonreassuring fetal heart rate</u> pattern. The client has a <u>history of cocaine use</u> and has symptoms of <u>abruptio placentae</u>.

D. G2 P1 at <u>42 weeks</u> who will give birth vaginally after <u>induced</u> labor. The client has been pushing for 2 hours, and <u>forceps</u> will be used.

likely to be meconium-stained

Complications of Childbearing

Chronic Hypertension

■ Hypertension and/or proteinuria in pregnant woman with chronic hypertension before 20 weeks of gestation and persistent after 12 weeks postpartum

A client at 33 weeks' gestation who has been diagnosed with pregnancy-induced hypertension (PIH) is admitted to the labor and delivery area. She is obviously nervous and expresses concern for the health of her baby. How should the nurse respond?

A. "You have the best doctor on the staff, so don't worry about a thing."

B. "Your anxiety is contributing to your condition and may be the reason for your admission."

C. "This is a minor problem that is easily controlled, and everything will be all right."

D. "As I assess you and your baby, I will explain the plan for your care and answer your questions."

Superimposed Pre-eclampsia or Eclampsia

■ Development of pre-eclampsia or eclampsia in woman with chronic hypertension before 20 weeks of gestation

Pre-eclampsia/Eclampsia

HELLP syndrome: Extremely severe form of gestational hypertension: **H**emolysis, **E**levated **L**iver Enzymes, **L**ow **P**latelets

■ Pre-eclampsia symptoms
  — BP
    • Mild: 30 mmHg systolic and/or 15 mmHg diastolic over baseline
    • Severe: Same (some sources say 160/110 mmHg × 2 or more)
  — Protein
    • Mild: >1+
    • Severe: 3+ to 4+

HESI Test Question Approach			
Positive?		YES	NO
Key Words			
Rephrase			
Rule Out Choices			
A	B	C	D

HESI Test Question Approach			
Positive?		YES	NO
Key Words			
Rephrase			
Rule Out Choices			
A	B	C	D

— Edema
  • Mild: Eyes, face, fingers
  • Severe: Generalized edema
— Deep tendon reflexes (DTRs)
  • Mild: May be normal
  • Severe: 3+ or more and clonus
— Central nervous system (CNS) symptoms
  • Mild: Headache, irritability
  • Severe: Severe headache, visual disturbances
— Other
  • Weight gain >2 lb/week
  • Oliguria (<100 mL/4 hr); epigastric pain related to liver enlargement
  • Elevated serum creatinine, thrombocytopenia, marked SGOT elevation

Nursing Interventions: Pre-eclampsia

■ Control stimulation in room
■ Explain procedures
■ Maintain IV (16- to 18-g venocatheter)
■ Monitor BP every 15 to 30 minutes and DTRs and urine for protein every 1 hour
■ Administer magnesium sulfate as prescribed ——————→ *prevention of seizures*
  lower BP
  sedation
■ Monitor magnesium levels and for signs of toxicity (urinary output <30 mL/hr, R <12 breaths/min, DTRs absent, deceleration of FHR, bradycardia)

Nursing Interventions: Eclampsia (Seizures)

■ Stay with client
■ Turn client on her side
■ Do not attempt to force objects into client's mouth
■ Administer O$_2$ and have suction available
■ Give magnesium sulfate as prescribed
■ Remember that seizures can occur postpartum   *grand mal seizures*
■ Magnesium sulfate is not an antihypertensive; it is used to prevent/control seizure. Withhold if any of the following is present:
  — R <12 breaths/min
  — Absent deep tendon reflexes (DTRs)
  — Urine output <30 mL/hr
■ Ensure that calcium gluconate 1g (10 ml of 10% solution) is available for emergency administration to reverse magnesium sulfate toxicity

Gestational Diabetes
Screening

■ Recommendations for glucose screening for all pregnant women
  — 1-hour glucose screen between 24 and 26 weeks
  — Goal is strict blood glucose control.
  — Oral glucose-lowering agents and insulin
    • Generally, Glyburide or insulin is used during pregnancy. Insulin does not cross the placenta, and glyburide only minimally crosses it.
    • Only regular insulin is used during labor because it is short acting, which makes it easier to maintain the mother's glucose level at 3.3–5.6 mmol/L (60 to 100 mg/dL).

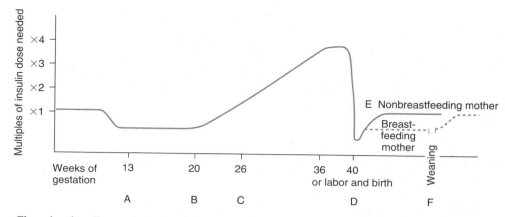

Figure 10-1 Changing insulin needs during pregnancy. (From Lowdermilk D, Perry S, Cashion K, Alden KR: *Maternity and women's health care,* ed 10, St Louis, 2012, Mosby.)

A client who has gestational diabetes asks the nurse to explain why her baby is at risk for macrosomia. Which explanation should the nurse offer?

A. The placenta receives decreased maternal blood flow during pregnancy because of vascular constriction.

B. The fetus secretes insulin in response to maternal hyperglycemia, causing weight gain and growth.

C. Infants of diabetic mothers are postmature, which allows the fetus extra time to grow.

D. Rapid fetal growth contributes to congenital anomalies, which are more common in infants of diabetic mothers.

glucose crosses placenta, but insulin does not

Preterm Labor (PTL)

■ Signs and symptoms of PTL
  — More than five contractions in an hour
  — Menstrual-like cramps
  — Low, dull backache
  — Pelvic pressure
  — Increase/change in vaginal discharge
  — Leaking or gush of amniotic fluid

Tocolytics and Their Administration

Tocolytics stop uterine contractions.

■ **Ritodrine (Yutopar)**
  — Side effects
    • Nervousness and tremulousness
    • Headache
    • N/V, diarrhea, epigastric pain
  — Adverse effects
    • Tachycardia
    • Chest pain with pulmonary edema
    • Low K⁺, hyperglycemia
  — Nursing interventions
    • Maternal ECG and lab tests
    • Cardiac and fetal monitoring
    • VS every 15 minutes
  — Antidote
    • Propranolol (Inderal)

HESI Test Question Approach			
Positive?		**YES**	**NO**
Key Words			
Rephrase			
Rule Out Choices			
A	B	C	D

get off feet
drink water
time contractions

133

- **Terbutaline (Brethine)**
  — Side effects
    - Nervousness and tremulousness
    - Headache
    - N/V, diarrhea, epigastric pain
  — Adverse effects
    - Tachycardia
    - Chest pain with pulmonary edema
    - Low K^+, hyperglycemia
  — Nursing interventions
    - Notify healthcare provider if the woman exhibits the following:
      □ Maternal heart rate greater than 130 beats/min; arrhythmias, chest pain
      □ BP less than 90/60 mm Hg
      □ Signs of pulmonary edema (e.g., dyspnea, crackles, decreased SaO_2)
      □ Fetal heart rate greater than 180 beats/min
    - Hyperglycemia occurs more frequently in women who are being treated simultaneously with corticosteroids
    - Ensure that the antidote: propranolol (Inderal) is available to reverse adverse effects related to cardiovascular function
    - Monitor I & O
    - Check weight daily
  — Antidote
    - Propranolol (Inderal)
- **Magnesium sulfate**
  — Side effects
    - CNS depression
    - Slowed respirations
    - Decreased DTRs
  — Adverse effects
    - Decreased urine output
    - Pulmonary edema
  — Nursing interventions
    - Hold if:
      □ Respirations < 12 breaths/min
      □ Urine output < 100 mL/4 hr
      □ Absent DTRs
    - Monitor serum magnesium levels - with higher doses; therapeutic range is between 4 and 7.5 mEq/L or 5-8 mg/dl
  — Antidote
    - Ensure that calcium gluconate 1 g (10 ml of 10% solution) is available for emergency administration to reverse magnesium sulfate toxicity
- **Drugs used to decrease contractions**
  — Indomethacin (Indocin)
  — channel bocker—Nifedipine (Procardia), nitroglycerin
- **Betamethasone** (Celestone) is used in PTL to enhance surfactant production and fetal lung maturity if the fetus is < 35 weeks of gestation

emotional needs [handwritten annotation pointing to A and B]

A client at 15 weeks' gestation is admitted for an inevitable abortion. Thirty minutes after returning from surgery, her vital signs are stable. Which nursing intervention has the highest priority?

A. Ask the client if she would like to talk about losing her baby

B. Place cold cabbage leaves on the client's breasts to reduce breast engorgement

C. Send a referral to the grief counselor for at-home follow-up

(D.) Confirm the client's Rh and Coombs status and administer RhoGAM (WinRho) if indicated.

✱Remember Maslow's hierarchy [handwritten annotation]

<table>
<tr><th colspan="4">HESI Test Question Approach</th></tr>
<tr><td>Positive?</td><td></td><td>YES</td><td>NO</td></tr>
<tr><td colspan="4">Key Words</td></tr>
<tr><td colspan="4"></td></tr>
<tr><td colspan="4"></td></tr>
<tr><td colspan="4">Rephrase</td></tr>
<tr><td colspan="4"></td></tr>
<tr><td colspan="4"></td></tr>
<tr><td colspan="4">Rule Out Choices</td></tr>
<tr><td>A</td><td>B</td><td>C</td><td>D</td></tr>
</table>

Miscarriage

Nursing Assessment

- Vaginal bleeding with a gestational age of 20 weeks or less
- Uterine cramping, backache, and pelvic pressure
- Maybe symptoms of shock
- Assess client/family emotional status, needs, and support

Nursing Interventions

- Monitor VS, LOC, and amount of bleeding
- Prepare client to receive IV fluids and/or blood
- If client is Rh negative, give RhoGAM (WinRho)

Incompetent Cervix

Incompetent cervix (recurrent premature dilation of the cervix) is passive, painless dilation of the cervix during the second trimester.

- Conservative management
  — Bed rest
  — Hydration
  — Tocolysis (inhibition of uterine contractions)
- Cervical cerclage may be performed.
  — McDonald cerclage: Band of homologous fascia or nonabsorbable ribbon (Mersilene) may be placed around the cervix beneath the mucosa to constrict the internal os of the cervix.
  — Cerclage procedure can be classified according to time or whether it is elective (prophylactic), urgent, or emergent.

Ectopic Pregnancy

Nursing Assessment

- Missed period but early signs of pregnancy absent
- Positive pregnancy test result
- Rupture
  — Sharp, unilateral pelvic pain
  — Vaginal bleeding
  — Referred shoulder pain
  — Syncope can lead to shock

Nursing Interventions

- Monitor hemodynamic status
- Prepare client for surgery and IV fluid administration, including blood

Abruptio Placentae and Placenta Previa

- **Abruptio Placentae**
  - Concealed or overt bleeding
  - Uterine tone ranges from tense without relaxation to tense and board-like
  - Persistently painful
  - Abnormal fetal heart rate - - Nonreassuring fetal heart rate pattern (the more area abrupted, the worse the FHR)
- **Placenta Previa**
  - Bright red vaginal bleeding
  - Soft uterine tone
  - Painless
  - FHR is normal unless bleeding is severe and mother becomes hypovolemic

If abruption or previa is suspected or confirmed, _no abdominal or vaginal manipulation_ such as:

- Leopold's maneuvers
- Vaginal examinations
- Internal monitor (especially if previa)
- Rectal examinations/enemas/suppositories

[handwritten margin note: contraindicated]

Disseminated Intravascular Coagulation

- Risk factors for DIC in pregnancy
  - Fetal demise
  - Infection/sepsis
  - Pregnancy-induced hypertension (pre-eclampsia)
  - Abruptio placentae

Dystocia

- A difficult birth resulting from problems involving the 5*P*s (powers, passage, passenger, psyche, and/or position); a lack of progress in cervical dilation, delay in fetal descent, or change in uterine contraction characteristics suggest dystocia.

Postpartum Infections

- Perineal infections
- Endometritis
- Parametritis
- Peritonitis
- Mastitis
- Deep vein thrombosis
- Cystitis
- Pyelonephritis
- HIV, hepatitis, other STIs
- Postpartum depression
  - Blues–emotionally labile from ~5-10 day postpartum–Reinforce need to rest, obtain support from family friends and community
  - Depression–occurs within 4 weeks of childbirth – irritability, ruminations of guilt and inadequacy – may have rejection of the infant. Supportive treatment including antidepressant agents and psychotherapy

[handwritten margin notes:]
Factors:
Preeclampsia
cocaine use
Cardiovascular &
renal problems
MVA & Trauma
→ detected by ultrasound

The nurse receives shift reports on four postpartum clients. Which client should the nurse assess first?

A. G3 P3, 7 hours after forceps delivery, who complains of pain and perineal pressure unrelieved by analgesics
B. G1 P1, 8 hours after cesarean delivery, who is receiving IV oxytocin (Pitocin) and complains of cramping with increased lochia when sitting
C. G2 P2, 5 hours after vaginal delivery, who complains of abdominal pain when the infant breast-feeds
D. G7 P6, 6 hours after vaginal delivery of twins, who reports saturating one pad in a 3-hour period

HESI Test Question Approach			
Positive?		YES	NO
Key Words			
Rephrase			
Rule Out Choices			
A	B	C	D

Which nursing action has the highest priority for an infant immediately after birth?

A. Place the infant's head in the "sniff" position and give oxygen via face mask
B. Perform a bedside glucose test and feed the infant glucose water as needed
C. Assess the heart rate and perform chest compressions if the heart rate is less than 60 beats/min
D. Dry the newborn and place the infant under a radiant warmer or skin-to-skin with the mother

HESI Test Question Approach			
Positive?		YES	NO
Key Words			
Rephrase			
Rule Out Choices			
A	B	C	D

Newborn Parameters (Approximate)

- Length: 18 to 22 inches
- Weight: 5.5 to 9.5 lb
- Head circumference: 13.2 to 14 inches
- Head should be one fourth the body length
- Sutures are palpable with fontanels
- Fontanel closure
  — Anterior: by 18 months
  — Posterior: 6 to 8 weeks
- Umbilical cord should have three vessels: two arteries and one vein
- Extremities should be flexed
- Major gluteal folds even
- Creases on soles of feet
- Ortolani's sign and Barlow's sign for developmental dysplasia of the hip
- Pulses palpable (radial, brachial, femoral)

Newborn Vital Signs

- Heart rate (resting): 100 to 160 beats/min (apical) by auscultating at the fourth intercostal space for 1 full minute
- Respirations: 30 to 60 breaths/min for 1 full minute
- Axillary temperature: 36° to 37.2° C (96.8° to 99° F)
- Blood pressure: 73/55 mmHg

Hypoglycemia

- Low blood glucose level
  - <1.7 mmol/L (30 mg/dL) in the first 72 hours of life
  - <2.5 mmol/L (35 mg/dL) after the first 3 days of life
- Normal blood glucose level
  - 1.7–3.3 mmol/L (30 to 60 mg/dL) in 1-day-old newborn
  - 2.2–5.0 mmol/L (40 to 90 mg/dL) in newborn > 1 day

Nursing Interventions

- Keep newborn warm
- Suction airway as necessary
- Observe for respiratory distress
- Normal or physiological jaundice appears after the first 24 hours in full-term newborns
- Pathological jaundice occurs before this time and may indicate early hemolysis of red blood cells
- Assess H & H and blood glucose levels
- Weigh daily
- Monitor I & O; weigh diapers if necessary (1 g = 1 mL of urine)
- Monitor temperature
- Observe for any cracks in the skin
- Administer eye medication within 1 hour after birth
- Provide cord care
- Provide circumcision care and teach client how to care for circumcision site
- Position newborn on right side after feeding; however, the side-lying position is not recommended for sleep, because this position makes it easy for the newborn to roll to the prone position
- Observe for normal stool and passage of meconium
- Test newborn's reflexes

Reflexes Exhibited and Age Reflexes Disappear

- Sucking or rooting: 3-4 months
- Moro: 3-4 months
- Tonic neck or fencing: 3-4 months
- Babinski's sign: 1 year–18 months
- Palmar-plantar grasp: 8 months
- Stepping or walking: 3-4 months

Major Newborn Complications

Respiratory Distress Syndrome

- Caused inability to produce surfactant
- Resulting in hypoxia and acidosis

Meconium Aspiration Syndrome

- Fetal distress increases intestinal peristalsis
- Releasing meconium into the amniotic fluid

Retinopathy of Prematurity

- Vascular disorder of retina
- Caused by the use of oxygen (>30 days)

high levels of O₂ can be toxic

Hyperbilirubinemia

- Jaundice becomes visible when the total serum bilirubin (TSB) reaches 85 mcmol/L (5 to 6 mg/dL)
- Jaundice is considered abnormal or nonphysiologic when TSB rises more rapidly and to higher levels than is expected or stays elevated for longer than normal
- Prevention of kernicterus, which results in permanent neurological damage
- Jaundice starts at head, spreads to chest, abdomen, arms, legs, hands, and feet
- Phototherapy: Use of fluorescent lights to reduce serum bilirubin levels
  - Possible adverse effects: Eye damage, dehydration, sensory deprivation
  - Expose as much of the skin as possible but cover genital area
  - Cover the eyes with eye shields
  - Monitor skin temperature closely
  - Increase fluids to compensate for water loss
  - Expect loose green stools and green urine
  - Monitor newborn's skin color
  - Reposition every 2 hours
  - Provide stimulation
  - After treatment, continue monitoring for signs of rebound hyperbilirubinemia

greatest concern is 7|2 mg/dL

ensure adequate hydration

Erythroblastosis Fetalis

- Destruction of red blood cells as a result of an antigen-antibody reaction
- Characterized by hemolytic anemia or hyperbilirubinemia
- Exchange of fetal and maternal blood occurs at birth; antibodies are harmless to the mother but cause fetal hemolysis
- Administer Rh-immune globulin (WinRho)
- Newborn's blood is replaced with Rh-negative blood to stop destruction of newborn's red blood cells
- Rh-negative blood gradually is replaced with newborn's own blood

occurs when mom is not given Rhogam

Sepsis

- Presence of bacteria in the blood

TORCH Infections

- Infections involving one of the following:
  - **T**oxoplasmosis
  - **O**ther infections (e.g., gonorrhea, syphilis, varicella, hepatitis B, HIV, or human parvovirus B19)
  - **R**ubella
  - **C**ytomegalovirus
  - **H**erpes simplex virus

Addicted Newborn

- Passive addiction to drugs that have passed through the placenta

CIWA → withdrawal symptoms

Fetal Alcohol Syndrome
- Caused by maternal alcohol use during pregnancy
- Causes mental and physical retardation

Newborn of a Mother with HIV
- Monitor antibody closely throughout pregnancy

Newborn of a Mother with Diabetes
- Infant born to mother with type 1 or type 2 diabetes or gestational diabetes
- Newborn may have hypoglycemia, hyperbilirubinemia, respiratory distress syndrome, hypocalcemia, birth trauma, and congenital anomalies

A pregnant client tells the nurse that she smokes only a few cigarettes a day. What information should the nurse provide the client about the effects of smoking during pregnancy?

A. Smoking causes vasoconstriction and reduces placental perfusion.
B. Smoking reduces the L:S ratio, contributing to lung immaturity.
C. Smoking causes vasodilation and increased fluid overload for the fetus.
D. Smoking during pregnancy places the fetus at risk for lung cancer.

HESI Test Question Approach		
Positive?	**YES**	**NO**
Key Words		
Rephrase		
Rule Out Choices		
A	B	C	D

Nurse-Client Relationship

- The goal of the nurse-client relationship is to help the client to develop problem-solving coping mechanisms.
- **Privacy and confidentiality:** A client's reasonable expectation that information revealed to the nurse will not be disclosed to others. However, the nurse must explain to the client that information relevant to the individual's treatment plan must be shared with the other members of the treatment team, especially if the client has thoughts of harming himself or herself or others.

Therapeutic Communication

- Both verbal and nonverbal expression
- Goal directed
- Appropriate, efficient, flexible, and elicits feedback
- Basic communication principles can be applied to all clients:
  - Establish trust
  - Demonstrate a nonjudgmental attitude
  - Offer self; be empathetic, not sympathetic
  - Use active listening
  - Accept and support client's feelings
  - Clarify and validate client's statements
  - Use matter-of-fact approach
- Examples of therapeutic communication
  - Silence: sit quietly and wait. Silence is planned
  - Active listening: gives full attention to the client
  - Open ended questioning: promotes sharing
  - Empathizing: demonstrating warmth and acknowledgment of feelings
  - Restating: repeats what the client says to show understanding and to review what was said.

Mental Health

- Mental health is a lifelong process of successful adjustment to changing environments (internal and external).

Mental Health Illness

- Mental health illness is the loss of the ability to respond to the environment in accord with oneself and society.

An adult client is admitted to the in-client mental health unit for severe depression. Although the client has agreed to electroconvulsive therapy (ECT), the client's partner states, "I'm concerned that his neurons will be destroyed by this treatment." Which response by the nurse is most helpful?

A. "I'll contact the nurse supervisor for you."
B. "Let's tour the ECT room and speak to the staff."
C. "I think you should show support for your partner.
D. "May we sit and discuss your concerns about ECT?"

ECT can affect short-term memory.

HESI Test Question Approach			
Positive?		YES	NO
Key Words			
Rephrase			
Rule Out Choices			
A	B	C	D

A female client who has just learned that she has breast cancer tells her family that the biopsy was negative. What action should the nurse take?

A. Remind the client that the results were positive
B. Ask the client to restate what the healthcare provider told her
C. Talk to the family about the client's need for family support
D. Encourage the client to talk to the nurse about her fears

HESI Test Question Approach			
Positive?		YES	NO
Key Words			
Rephrase			
Rule Out Choices			
A	B	C	D

Coping and Defense Mechanisms

- Efforts to reduce anxiety
- Can be constructive or destructive
- *Coping* is related to problem solving
- *Defense* is related to protecting oneself
  — *Examples:* Denial, displacement, identification

Treatment Modalities

- *Milieu therapy:* The physical and social environment in which the client is receiving treatment
- *Interpersonal psychotherapy:* Uses a therapeutic relationship to modify the client's feelings, attitudes, and behaviors
- *Behavior therapy:* Takes many forms and is used to change the client's behaviors
- *Cognitive therapy:* Directive, time-limited approach
- *Crisis intervention:* Directed at resolution of the immediate crisis and to returning the individual to the precrisis level of functioning
- *Electroconvulsive therapy (ECT):* The use of electrically induced seizures to treat severely depressed individuals who fail to respond to antidepressant medications and therapy

142

The nurse is facilitating a support group for stress management. During the initial phase, a female group member states that she can help the group more because she has a master's degree. How should the nurse respond?

A. Restate the purpose of the support group sessions
B. Ask the group to identify various stressful problems
C. Obtain ideas from the members about strategies for stressful situations
D. Conclude the meeting and evaluate the session

HESI Test Question Approach			
Positive?		**YES**	**NO**
Key Words			
Rephrase			
Rule Out Choices			
A	**B**	**C**	**D**

Group Therapy

- Involves a therapist and five to eight members
- Provides feedback and support for the individual goals *eye contact* of each member
- Group therapy models
  — Psychoanalytical
  — Transactional analysis
  — Rogerian therapy
  — Gestalt therapy
- Interpersonal group therapy
- Self-help or support groups
- Family therapy
  — The member with the presenting symptoms indicates the presence of problems in the entire family.
  — A change in one member brings about changes in other members.

Stages of Group Development

- Initial stage: Superficial communication
- Working stage: Real work is done by group
- Termination stage: Provides opportunity to learn to deal with letting go

The nurse and the UAP takes a group of mental health clients to a baseball game. During the game, a male client begins to complain of shortness of breath and dizziness. Which intervention should the nurse implement first?

A. Send the client back to the unit
B. Ask for a description of his feelings
C. Escort the client to a quiet area
D. Inquire about what is most stressful

HESI Test Question Approach			
Positive?		**YES**	**NO**
Key Words			
Rephrase			
Rule Out Choices			
A	**B**	**C**	**D**

Anxiety

Anxiety is a normal subjective experience that includes feeling of apprehension, uneasiness, uncertainty, or dread.

Types of Anxiety
- *Mild:* Tension of everyday life
- *Moderate:* Immediate concerns
- *Severe:* Feeling that something bad is about to happen
- *Panic:* Terror and a sense of impending doom

Anxiety Disorders
Generalized Anxiety Disorder
- Unrealistic anxiety about everyday worries
- Panic disorders—produce a sudden feeling of intense apprehension

Posttraumatic Stress Disorder
- Individual re-experiences traumatic event
- Recurrent and intrusive dreams or flashbacks

Phobias
- Irrational fear of an object, activity, or situation
- Client may recognize fear as unreasonable
- Associated with panic-level anxiety
- Defense mechanisms include repression and displacement

Nursing Interventions
- Reduce stimuli in the environment
- Provide a calm, quiet environment
- Administer antianxiety medications as prescribed
- Administer SSRIs and tricyclic antidepressants as prescribed

The nurse is planning to teach a male client strategies for coping with his anxiety. The nurse finds him in his room, compulsively washing his hands. What action should the nurse take next?
A. Teach him alternatives as he washes his hands
B. Ask him to stop his hand washing immediately
C. Allow him to finish hand washing before teaching
D. Ask what precipitated the hand washing

HESI Test Question Approach		
Positive?	YES	NO
Key Words		
Rephrase		
Rule Out Choices		

A	B	C	D

Obsessive-Compulsive Disorder
- *Obsessions:* Persistently intrusive thoughts
- *Compulsions:* Repetitive behaviors designed to divert unacceptable thought and reduce anxiety

Antianxiety (Anxiolytic) Medications
- These drugs depress the CNS
  - **Benzodiazepines** have anxiety-reducing (anxiolytic), sedative-hypnotic, muscle-relaxing, and anticonvulsant actions.
  - **Flumazenil** (Anexate [Canada]; Romazicon), a benzodiazepine antagonist administered intravenously, reverses benzodiazepine intoxication in 5 minutes.

Somatic Symptom Disorder
Persistent worry or complaints about physical illness without physical findings.
- Types of somatoform disorders
  - Conversion disorder
  - Hypochondriasis
  - Somatization disorders
- Treatment: Cognitive behavioral therapy

The nurse is talking to a client with a dissociative identity disorder. During the interaction, the client begins to dissociate. Which action should the nurse take?
A. Escort the client to art therapy group
B. Call the client by name
C. Talk about stressful feelings
D. Move to another setting

HESI Test Question Approach			
Positive?		YES	NO
Key Words			
Rephrase			
Rule Out Choices			
A	B	C	D

Crisis Intervention
- A crisis results from the experiencing of a significant traumatic event or situation that cannot be remedied by the use of available coping strategies
- Risk factors include multiple comorbidities, multiple losses, unexpected life changes, limited coping skills, chronic pain or disability, poor social support, concurrent psychiatric disorders, substance abuse or disability and limited access to health care service
- Goal is to return client to pre-crisis level of functioning

Nursing Interventions

- Assess for suicidal or homicidal thoughts or plans
- Help client feel safe and less anxious
- Listen carefully
- Be directive (e.g., nurse may arrange for shelter or contact a social worker)
- Mobilize social support
- Involve client in identifying realistic, acceptable interventions
- Plan regular follow-up

Dissociative Disorders

These disorders are associated with exposure to an extremely traumatic event.

- *Dissociative amnesia:* One or more episodes of inability to recall important personal information, usually of a traumatic nature.
- *Dissociative fugue:* Sudden, unexpected travel away from home, with an inability to recall one's past.
- *Dissociative identity disorder:* Two or more distinct identities, at least two of which recurrently take control.
- *Depersonalization disorder:* Persistent or recurrent episodes of feelings of detachment from oneself.

Personality Disorders

- Inflexible maladaptive behavior patterns
- In touch with reality
- Lack of insight into one's behavior
- Forms of acting out
  - Yelling and swearing
  - Cutting oneself
  - Manipulation
  - Substance abuse
  - Promiscuous sexual behaviors
  - Suicide attempts

Cluster A (Odd and Eccentric)

- Paranoid
- Schizoid
- Schizotypal

Cluster B (Emotional and Dramatic)

- Antisocial (withdrawn)
- Borderline (low self-esteem)
- Histrionic (emotionally immature)
- Narcissistic (always right)

Cluster C (Anxious and Tense)

- Avoidant (sensitive to rejection)
- Dependent (whining behavior, feel inadequate)
- Obsessive-compulsive (rigid; must be done a certain way)

A female client who has borderline personality disorder returns after a weekend pass with lacerations to both wrists. The client whines and complains to the nurse during the dressing change. The tone of the nurse's response should be:

A. Distant
B. Concerned
C. Matter of fact
D. Empathetic

HESI Test Question Approach			
Positive?		YES	NO
Key Words			
Rephrase			
Rule Out Choices			
A	B	C	D

Eating Disorders

Compulsive Overeating

- Bingelike overeating without purging
- Lack of control over food consumption

Anorexia Nervosa

- Onset often associated with a stressful event
- Death can occur from starvation, suicide, cardiomyopathies, or electrolyte imbalance
- Client experiences an altered body image

Bulimia Nervosa

- Binge-purge syndrome in which eating binges are followed by purging behaviors.

A client with bulimia is admitted to the mental health unit. What intervention is most important for the nurse to include in the initial treatment plan?

A. Observe the client after meals for vomiting
B. Assess daily weight and vital signs
C. Monitor serum potassium and calcium
D. Provide a structured environment at mealtime

HESI Test Question Approach			
Positive?		YES	NO
Key Words			
Rephrase			
Rule Out Choices			
A	B	C	D

The mental health RN is assigned to four clients. Which client should be assessed first?

- (A.) A newly admitted client diagnosed with major depression whose assessment is incomplete
- B. A client with schizophrenia who is having auditory hallucinations of someone crying
- C. A client who recently became unemployed and has a 10-year history of daily alcohol use
- D. A client with anorexia nervosa having difficulty attending group therapy

HESI Test Question Approach			
Positive?		YES	NO
Key Words			
Rephrase			
Rule Out Choices			
A	B	C	D

| Mood Disorders

Depression

- Characterized by feelings of hopelessness, low self-esteem, self-blame
- 25% of those with depression have suicidal ideation
- Behavior therapy, cognitive behavioral therapy, and interpersonal psychotherapy
- Antidepressant Medication Therapy
  — Cyclic antidepressants (e.g., TCAs)
  — SSRIs and SNRIs
  — Atypical antidepressants

Suicide

Suicide threat is a warning, direct or indirect, verbal or nonverbal, that a person is planning to take his or her own life. The person may give away prized possessions, make a will or funeral arrangements, or withdraw from friendships and social activities. Assessment includes whether the person has made a specific plan and whether the means to carry out the plan are available.

Nursing Interventions

- NEVER leave a suicidal client alone
- Protect the client from inflicting harm, be vigilant, supervise medication administration, implement strategies to ↑ self-esteem and social support
- Be aware of major warning signs of impending attempt
  — Client begins to give away possessions
  — Client becomes "better" or "happy"!

Bipolar Disorder

- Characterized by episodes of mania and depression with periods of normal mood and activity in between
- Lithium carbonate is the medication of choice; it can be toxic and requires regular monitoring of serum lithium levels
- Other medications
  — Divalproex (Depakote; Valproate)
  — Olanzapine (Zyprexa)
  — Carbamazepine (Tegretol)

Lithium:
0.8-1.2
Draw twice/week until stabilized
muscle weakness
confusion
seizures

Other Therapy:
non-competitive exercise
finger foods

Purpose of Antidepressants

Antidepressants have been approved for depression, phobias, eating disorders, and anxiety disorders.

Monoamine Oxidase Inhibitors (MAOIs)

- Inhibit the enzyme monoamine oxidase, which is present in the brain, blood platelets, liver, spleen, and kidneys
- Administered to clients with depression who have not responded to other antidepressant therapies, including electroconvulsive therapy
- Concurrent use with amphetamines, antidepressants, dopamine, epinephrine, guanethidine, levodopa, methyldopa, nasal decongestants, norepinephrine, reserpine, tyramine-containing foods, or vasoconstrictors may cause hypertensive crisis
- Concurrent use with opioid analgesics may cause hypertension or hypotension, coma, or seizures

Nursing Implications and Client Education

- Selective serotonin reuptake inhibitors (SSRIs)
  — Inhibit serotonin uptake
- Tricyclic antidepressants (TCAs)
  — Block the reuptake of norepinephrine (and serotonin) at the presynaptic neuron
  — May take several weeks to produce the desired effect (2 to 4 weeks after the first dose)

Schizophrenia

- A group of mental disorders characterized by psychotic features
  — *Delusions of persecution:* Client believes he or she is being persecuted by some powerful force
  — *Delusions of grandeur:* Client has an exaggerated sense of self that has no basis in reality
  — *Somatic delusions:* Client believes his or her body is changing, with no basis in reality
- Perceptual distortions
  — *Illusions:* Brief experiences of misinterpretation or misperception of reality
  — *Hallucinations* (five senses): false perceptions with no basis in reality
    - Safety is the first priority. Make sure client does not have an auditory command telling him or her to harm himself or herself or others.

Nursing interventions

- Assess for risk of violence to self or others and take appropriate precautions
- Provide quiet soothing environment
- Establish routine and boundaries
- Provide stable, nonthreatening, brief, social interactions
- If acting frightened or scared increase physical space surrounding client and approach calmly
- Encourage reality based interests

Antipsychotic Medications

- Traditional medications
  — Purpose
    - Treat psychotic behavior
  — Side effects
    - Extrapyramidal *(pill rolling, shuffling gait,*
    - Anticholinergic *(dry secretions)   etc.)*
  — *Nursing implications*
    - Encourage fluid (water)
    - Gum
    - Hard candy
    - Increase fiber intake
- Long-acting medications
  — Purpose
    - Promote medication compliance
  — Side effects
    - Blood dyscrasias
    - Neuroleptic malignant syndrome
  — *Nursing implications*
    - Change position slowly for dizziness
    - Report urinary retention to healthcare provider
- **Atypical medications**
  — Purpose
    - Treat all positive and negative symptoms
  — Side effects
    - Multiple side effects, depending on medication
  — *Nursing implications*
    - Tolerance to effects usually occurs

Neuroleptic malignant syndrome is a potentially fatal condition that may occur at any time during therapy with neuroleptic (antipsychotic) medications.

Substance Abuse Disorders

- *Substance dependence:* A pattern of repeated use of a substance
- *Substance tolerance:* A need for more of the substance to reach the desired effect
- *Substance abuse:* Recurrent use of a substance
- *Substance withdrawal:* The occurrence of symptoms when blood levels of a substance decline

Alcohol Abuse
Alcohol is a central nervous system (CNS) depressant.
- *Physical dependence:* A biological need for alcohol to avoid physical withdrawal symptoms
- *Psychological dependence:* A craving for the subjective effect of alcohol
- *Intoxication:* Blood alcohol level $\geq$ 0.1% (21.7 mmol/L [100 mg alcohol/dL] blood)

Alcohol Withdrawal
- Signs peak after 24 to 48 hours.
- Chlordiazepoxide (Librium) is the most commonly prescribed medication for acute alcohol withdrawal.

(handwritten note:) NB NMS:
Fever
Autonomic changes
Rigidity of muscles
Mental status changes

- Withdrawal delirium: Peaks 48 to 72 hours after cessation of intake and lasts 2 to 3 days.
  — **Medical emergency**
  — Death can occur from myocardial infarction, fat emboli, peripheral vascular collapse, electrolyte imbalance, aspiration pneumonia, or suicide.

Disulfiram (Antabuse) Therapy
- Alcohol deterrent
- Other medications used to assist with cravings
  — Acamprosate calcium (Campral)
  — Naltrexone (ReVia)
- Instruct client taking disulfiram to avoid the use of substances that contain alcohol, such as cough medicines, mouthwashes, and aftershave lotions.

A male client with a history of alcohol abuse is admitted to the medical unit for GI bleeding and pancreatitis. His admission data include: BP–156/96 mmHg, pulse–92 beats/min, and temp–37.3°C (99.2° F). Which intervention is most important for the nurse to implement?
A. Provide a quiet, low-stimulus environment
B. Initiate seizure precautions
C. Administer PRN lorazepam (Ativan) as prescribed
D. Determine the time and quantity of the client's last alcohol intake

Autism Spectrum Disorder
- Etiology—no known cause
- Clinical description
  — Hyperactivity
  — Short attention span
  — Impulsivity
  — Aggressivity
  — Self-injurious behavior
  — Temper tantrums
  — Repetitive mannerisms
  — Preoccupied with objects
  — Spoken language often absent
  — "Islands of genius"
- Prognosis: There is no cure for autism. Language skills and intellectual level are the strongest factors related to the prognosis. Only a small percentage of individuals with the disorder go on to live and work independently as adults.
- *Asperger's disorder* has many features similar to those of autism but does not show significant delays in language, cognitive development, age-appropriate self-help skills, adaptive behavior, or curiosity about the environment. It is a lifelong disorder.

HESI Test Question Approach			
Positive?		YES	NO
Key Words			
Rephrase			
Rule Out Choices			
A	B	C	D

Attention-Deficit/Hyperactivity Disorder

- Etiology—no known cause, but strong correlation with genetic factors
- Clinical description
  — Fidgeting in a seat
  — Getting up when expected to be seated
  — Excessive running when dangerous or inappropriate
  — Loud, disruptive play during quiet activities
  — Forgets and misses appointments
  — Fails to meet deadlines
  — Loses the train of conversation
  — Changes topics inappropriately
  — Does not follow rules of games
- Prognosis: Condition continues into adolescence in most children. Many adults who had ADHD in childhood report a decrease of hyperactivity but a continuation of difficulty concentrating or attending to complex projects.

Clients with ADHD may require CNS stimulants to reduce hyperactive behavior and lengthen attention span.

Dementia and Alzheimer's Disease

- Dementia is a syndrome of progressive deterioration in intellectual functioning secondary to structural or functional changes
- Marked by long-term and short-term memory loss
- Impairment in judgment, abstract thinking, problem-solving ability, and behavior also seen
- Most common type of dementia is Alzheimer's disease, an irreversible form of senile dementia caused by nerve cell deterioration
- Providing a safe environment is a priority in the care of clients with Alzheimer's disease; *calm environment*

maintain comfort
provide toileting & keep dry
provide soothing music
reassurance & companionship

Medications

- **Donepezil** (Aricept)
- **Galantamine** hydrobromide (Reminyl [Canada]; Razadyne)
- **Memantine** (Ebixia [Canada]; Namenda)
- **Rivastigmine** (Exelon)
- **Tacrine** (Cognex)

provides some time for cognitive stability.

Appendix A
Normal Laboratory Values

Test	Adult	Child	Infant/Newborn	Elder	Nursing Implications
Hematological					
Hgb (hemo-globin): mmol/L (g/dL)	Male: 140-180 (14-18) Female: 120-160 (12-16) Pregnant: >110 (>11)	1-6 yr: 95-140 (9.5-14) 6-18 yr: 100-150 (10-15.5)	Neonate (0-28 days): 140-240 (14-24) Newborn 1-2 months: 120-200 (12-20) 2-6 mo: 100-170 (10-17) 6 mo-1 yr: 95-140 (9.5-14)	Values slightly decreased	High-altitude living increases values. Drug therapy can alter values. Slight Hgb decreases normally occur during pregnancy.
Hct (hemato-crit): volume fraction (%)	Male: 0.42-0.52 volume frac-tion (42-52) Female: 0.37-0.47 volume fraction (37-47) Pregnant: >0.33 volume fraction (>33)	6-12 years: Male 0.31-0.38 (31-38) Female 0.32-0.39 (32-39) 12-18 years: Male 0.31-0.41 (31-41) Female 0.32-0.39 (32-39)	Newborn: Male 0.37-0.47 (37-47) Female 0.38-0.48 (38-48) 15-30 days: Male 0.41-0.43 (41-43) Female 0.34-0.42 (34-42) 61-180 days: Male 0.31-0.38 (31-38) Female 0.31-0.39 (31-39) 6 months to 2 years: Male 0.31-0.36 (31-36) Female 0.31-0.36 (31-36)	Values slightly decreased	Prolonged stasis from vaso-constriction secondary to the tourniquet can alter values. Abnormalities in RBC size may alter Hct values.
RBC (red blood cell) count: × 10¹²/L	Male: 4.7-6.1 Female: 4.2-5.4	1-6 yr: 4-5.5 6-18 yr: 4.5-5	Newborn: 4.8-7.1 2-8 wk: 4-6 2-6 mo: 3.5-5.5 6 mo-1yr: 3.5-5.2	Same as adult	Never draw a specimen from an arm with an infusing IV. Exercise and high altitudes can cause an increase in values. Values are usually lower during pregnancy. Drug therapy can alter values.
WBC (white blood cell) count: × 10⁹/L (mm³)	Both genders: 5-10 (5000-10,000)	≤2 yr: 6.2-17 (6200-17,000) ≥2 yr: 5-10 (5000-10,000)	Newborn (0-6 weeks) 9-30 (9000-30,000)	Same as adult	Anesthetics, stress, exercise, and convulsions can cause increased values. Drug therapy can decrease values. 24-48 hr postpartum: A count as high as 25,000 is normal.

(Continued)

Test	Adult	Child	Infant/Newborn	Elder	Nursing Implications
Hematological					
Platelet count: $\times 10^9$/L (mm³)	Both genders: 150-400 (150,000-400,000)	150-400 (150,000-400,000)	Premature infant: 100-300 (100,000-300,000) Newborn: 150-300 (150,000-300,000) Infant: 200-475 (200,000-475,000)	Same as adult	Living at high altitudes, exercising strenuously, or taking oral contraceptives may increase values. Decreased values may be caused by hemorrhage, DIC, reduced production of platelets, infections, use of prosthetic heart valves, and drugs (e.g., acetaminophen, aspirin, chemotherapy, H_2 blockers, INH, Levaquin, streptomycin, sulfonamides, thiazide diuretics).

HESI Hint: The laboratory values that are most important to know for the NCLEX-RN exam are Hgb, Hct, WBCs, Na+, K+, BUN, blood glucose, ABGs (arterial blood gases), bilirubin for newborns, and therapeutic range for PT and PTT.

Test	Adult	Child	Infant/Newborn	Elder	Nursing Implications
SED rate, ESR (erythrocyte sedimentation rate): mm/hr	Male: up to 15 Female: up to 20 Pregnant (all trimesters): up to 10	Same as adult	Newborn: 0-2	Same as adult	Pregnancy (second and third trimester) can cause elevations in ESR.
PT (prothrombin time): sec	Both genders: 11-12.5 Pregnant: slight ↓	Same as adult	Same as adult	Same as adult	PT is used to help regulate Coumadin dosages. Therapeutic range: 1.5 to 2 times normal or control.
PTT (partial thromboplastin time): sec (see APTT, below)	Both genders: 60-70 Pregnant: slight ↓	Same as adult	Same as adult	Same as adult	PTT is used to help regulate heparin dosages. Therapeutic range: 1.5 to 2.5 times normal or control.
INR (international normalized ratio)	Both genders: 0.8-1.2	Same as adult	Same as adult	Same as adult	Ideal INR value must be individualized. Typical values for certain clients are: Clients with atrial fibrillation and DVT: between 2.0 and 3.0 Clients with mechanical heart valves: between 3.0 and 4.0.
APTT (activated partial thromboplastin time): sec	Both genders: 30-40	Same as adult	Same as adult	Same as adult	APTT is used to help regulate heparin dosages. Therapeutic range: 1.5 to 2.5 times normal or control.

Test	Adult	Child	Infant/Newborn	Elder	Nursing Implications
Blood Chemistry					
Alkaline phosphatase: U/L	Both genders: 35-120	1-3 years: 185-383 4-6 years: 191-450 7-9 years: 218-499 10-11 years: Male 174-624 Female 169-657 12-13 years: Male 245-584 Female 141-499 14-15 years: Male 169-618 Female 103-283 16-19 years: Male 98-317 Female 82-169		Slightly higher than adult	Hemolysis of specimen can cause falsely elevated values.
Albumin: g/dL	Both genders: 35-50 (3.5-5) Pregnant: slight ↓	40-59 (4.5-9)	Premature infant: 30-42 (3-4.2) Newborn: 35-54 (3.5-5.4) Infant: 44-54 (4.4-5.4)	Same as adult	No special preparation is needed.
Bilirubin total: mcmol/L (mg/dL)	Total: 5.1-17 (0.3-1) Indirect: 3.4-12 (0.2-0.8) Direct: 1.7-5.1 (0.1-0.3)	Same as adult	Newborn: < 100 (1-12)	Same as adult	Client is kept NPO, except for water, for 8-12 hr before testing. Prevent hemolysis of blood during venipuncture. Do *not* shake tube; this can cause inaccurate values. Protect blood sample from bright light.
Hematological					
Calcium: mmol/L (mg/dL)	Both genders: 2.25-2.75 (9-10.5)	2.2-2.7 (8.8-10.8)	<10 days: 1.9-2.60 (7.6-10.4) Umbilical: 2.25-2.88 (9-11.5) 10 days-2 yr: 2.3-2.65 (9-10.6)	Values tend to decrease.	No special preparation is needed. Use of thiazide diuretics can cause increased calcium values.
Chloride: mmol/L (mEq/L)	Both genders: 98-106	90-110	Newborn: 96-106 Premature infant: 95-106	Same as adult	Do not collect from an arm with an infusing IV solution.
Cholesterol: mmol/L (mg/dL)	Both genders: <5.0 (<200)	10-11 years: Male 3.10-5.90 (120-228) Female 3.16-6.26 (122-242)	Infant (7-12 months): Male 2.15-5.30 (83-205) Female 1.76-5.59 (68-216) Newborn (0-1 month): Male 0.98-4.50 (38-174) Female 1.45-5.04 (56-195)	Same as adult	Do not collect from an arm with an infusing IV solution.

(Continued)

Test	Adult	Child	Infant/Newborn	Elder	Nursing Implications
			Hematological		
CPK (creatine phosphoki-nase): U/L	Male: 55-170 Female: 30-135	Same as adult	Newborn: 68-580	Same as adult	Specimen must not be stored before running test.
Creatinine: mcmol/L (mg/dL)	Male: 53-106 (0.6-1.2) Female: 44-97 (0.5-1.1)	Child/Adolescent (1-18 years): 18-62 (0.2-0.7)	Newborn (0-1 week): 53-97 (0.6-1.1) Infant (7 days-12 months): 18-35 (0.2-0.4)	Decrease in muscle mass may cause decreased values.	NPO for 8 hr before testing is preferred but not required. BUN-to-creatinine ratio of 20:1 indicates adequate kidney functioning.
Glucose: mmol/L (mg/dL)	Both genders: 4-6 (36-108)	≤2 yr: 3.3-5.5 (60-100) >2 yr: <6.1 (70-110)	Cord: 2.5-5.3 (45-96) Premature infant: 1.1-3.3 (20-60) Neonate (0-28 days): 1.7-3.3 (30-60) Infant (1 month-2 years): 2.2-5.0 (40-90)	Normal range increases after age 50.	Client is kept NPO, except for water, for 8 hr before testing. Stress, infection, and caffeine can cause increased values.
HCO_3^-: mmol/L (mEq/L)	Both genders: 21-28	21-28	Newborn/Infant: 16-24	Same as adult	None
Iron: mcmol/L (mcg/dL)	Male: 14-32 (80-180) Female: 11-29 (60-160)	Child 4-10 years: Male: 2.7-22.9 (15-128) Female: 5.0-21.8 (28-122)	Newborn: Male: 12.9-36.3 (72-203) Female: 13.4-42.1 (75-235)	Same as adult	NPO for 8 hr before test is preferred but not required.
TIBC (total iron binding capac-ity): mcmol/L (mcg/dL)	Both genders: 45-82 (250-460)	Same as adult	Newborn: 16.8-41.5 (94-232)	Same as adult	None
LDH (Lactate dehydroge-nase): U/L	Both genders: 100-190	60-170	Newborn: 160-450 Infant: 100-250	Same as adult	Do not give IM injections for 8-12 hr before test. Hemolysis of blood causes a false positive result.
Potassium: mmol/L (mEq/L)	Both genders: 3.5-5	3.4-4.7	Newborn: 3.9-5.9 Infant: 4.1-5.3	Same as adult	Hemolysis of specimen can result in falsely elevated values. Exercise of the forearm with tourniquet in place may cause an increased potassium level.
Protein total: g/L (g/dL)	Both genders: 64-83 (6.4-8.3)	62-80 (6.2-8)	Premature infant: 42-76 (4.2-7.6) Newborn: 46-74 (4.6-7.4) Infant: 60-67 (6-6.7)	Same as adult	NPO for 8 hr before test is preferred but not required.
AST/SGOT (aspartate ami-notransferase): U/L	0-35 Female slightly lower than adult male	3-6 yr: 15-50 6-12 yr: 10-50 12-18 yr: 10-40	0-5 days: 35-140 <3 yr: 15-60	Slightly higher than adult	Hemolysis of specimen can result in falsely elevated values. Exercise may cause an increased value.

(Continued)

Test	Adult	Child	Infant/Newborn	Elder	Nursing Implications
Hematological					
ALT/SGPT (alanine aminotransferase): U/mL	Both genders: 4-36	Child: 1-3 years: Male 19-59 Female 24-59 4-6 years: 24-49 14-15 years: Male 24-54 Female 19-44 16-19 years: Male 24-54 Female 19-49 U/L	Infant: 1-7 days: Male 6-40 Female 7-40 8-30 days: Male 10-40 Female 8-32 1-3 months: Male 13-39 Female 12-47 4-6 months: Male 12-42 Female 12-37 7-12 months: Male 13-45 Female 12-41	Slightly higher than adult	Hemolysis of specimen can result in falsely elevated values. Exercise may cause an increased value.
Sodium: mmol/L (mEq/L)	Both genders: 136-145	136-145	Newborn: 134-144 Infant: 134-150	Same as adult	Do not collect from an arm with an infusing IV solution.
Triglycerides: mg/dL	Male: 0.45-1.81 (40-160) Female: 0.40-1.52 (35-135)	4-6 years Male 0.36-1.31 (32-116) Female 0.36-1.31 (32-116) 7-9 years Male 0.32-1.46 (28-129) Female 0.32-1.46 (28-129) 10-11 Years Male 0.27-1.55 (24-137) Female 0.44-1.58 (39-140) 12-13 years Male 0.27-1.64 (24-145) Female 0.42-1.47 (37-130) 14-15 years Male 0.38-1.86 (34-165) Female 0.43-1.52 (38-135) 16-19 years Male 0.38-1.58 (34-140) Female 0.42-1.58 (37-140)	0-3 years : Male 0.31-1.41 (27-125) Female 0.31-1.41 (27-125)	Same as adult	Client is kept NPO for 12 hr before test. No alcohol for 24 hr before test.

(Continued)

Test	Adult	Child	Infant/Newborn	Elder	Nursing Implications
Hematological					
BUN (blood urea nitrogen): mmol/L (mg/dL)	Both genders: 3.6-7.1 (10-20)	1.8-6.4 (5-18)	Newborn: 0.7-4.6 (2-13) Cord: 7.5-14.3 (21-40) Infant: 1.8-6.0 (5-17)	Slightly higher	None
Arterial Blood Chemistry					
pH	Both genders: 7.35-7.45	Child > 2 years: Same as adult	Newborn: 7.32-7.49 2 months-2 years: 7.34-7.46	Same as adult	Specimen must be heparinized. Specimen must be iced for transport. All air bubbles must be expelled from sample. Direct pressure to puncture site must be maintained.
Pco_2: mmHg	Both genders: 35-45	Same as adult	<2 yr: 26-41	Same as adult	Specimen must be heparinized. Specimen must be iced for transport. All air bubbles must be expelled from sample. Direct pressure to puncture site must be maintained.
Po_2: mmHg	Both genders: 80-100	Same as adult	Newborn: 60-70	Same as adult	Specimen must be heparinized. Specimen must be iced for transport. All air bubbles must be expelled from sample. Direct pressure to puncture site must be maintained.
Hco_3^-: mmol/L (mEq/L)	Both genders: 21-28	Same as adult	Newborn/Infant: 16-24	Same as adult	Specimen must be heparinized. Specimen must be iced for transport. All air bubbles must be expelled from sample. Direct pressure to puncture site must be maintained.
O_2 Saturation: %	Both genders: 95-100	Same as adult	Newborn: 40-90	95	Specimen must be heparinized. Specimen must be iced for transport. All air bubbles must be expelled from sample. Direct pressure to puncture site must be maintained.

From Pagana TJ, Pagana KD: *Mosby's Canadian Manual of Diagnostic and Laboratory Test*, 1st ed, Toronto, 2013, Mosby.

From Pagana TJ, Pagana KD: Mosby's Manual of Diagnostic and Laboratory Test, 11th ed, St. Louis, 2013, Mosby.

BUN, Blood urea nitrogen; *DIC,* disseminated intravascular coagulation; *DVT,* deep vein thrombosis; *IM,* intramuscular; *INH,* isoniazid; *NPO,* nothing by mouth; *Pco₂,* carbon dioxide partial pressure; *Po₂,* oxygen partial pressure; *Hco₃⁻,* bicarbonate.

Appendix B
Comparison of Three Types of Hepatitis

Characteristics	Hepatitis A (Infectious Hepatitis)	Hepatitis B (Serum Hepatitis)	Hepatitis C
Source of infection	• Contaminated food • Contaminated water or shellfish	• Contaminated blood products • Contaminated needles or surgical instruments • Mother to child at birth	• Contaminated blood products • Contaminated needles, IV drug use • Dialysis
Route of infection	• Oral • Fecal • Parenteral • Person to person	• Parenteral • Oral • Fecal • Direct contact • Breast milk • Sexual contact	• Parenteral • Sexual contact
Incubation period	15-50 days	14-180 days	14-180 days (average)
Onset	Abrupt	Insidious	Insidious
Seasonal variation	• Autumn • Winter	All year	All year
Age group affected	• Children • Young adults	Any age	Any age
Vaccine	Yes	Yes	No
Inoculation	Yes	Yes	Yes
Potential for chronic liver disease	No	Yes	Yes
Immunity	Yes	Yes	No
Treatment	• Prevention—Hepatitis A (HAV) vaccine • Proper hand washing • Avoid contaminated food or water • Obtain immunoglobulin within 14 days if exposed to the virus	• Prevention—Hepatitis B (HBV) vaccine for high-risk groups • Antiviral and immunomodulating drugs	• Subcutaneous pegylated interferon alpha once a week and oral ribavirin (Copegus, Rebetol) daily
Complications	Very few	• Chronic hepatitis • Cirrhosis • Hepatitis D • Liver cancer	• Chronic hepatitis • Cirrhosis • Liver cancer

NCLEX-RN Examination Practice Questions

Management/Leadership

1. **Which activity should the nurse delegate to an unlicensed assistive personnel (UAP)?**
   A. Check to see whether a client with cirrhosis can hear any better after discontinuation of an IV antibiotic
   B. Encourage additional PO fluids for an elderly client with pneumonia who has developed a fever
   C. Report the ability of a client with myasthenia gravis to manage the supper tray independently
   D. Record the number of liquid stools of a client who received lactulose for an elevated NH_3 level

HESI Test Question Approach		
Positive?	**YES**	**NO**
Key Words		
Rephrase		
Rule Out Choices		
A	B	C	D

2. **The nurse is assigning clients to the UAP. Which client requires intervention by the RN?**
   A. The client with active TB who is leaving the room without a mask
   B. The client with dehydration who is requesting something to drink
   C. The client with asthma who complains of being anxious and cannot concentrate
   D. The client with COPD who is leaving the unit to smoke, even though the next IVPB is due

HESI Test Question Approach		
Positive?	**YES**	**NO**
Key Words		
Rephrase		
Rule Out Choices		
A	B	C	D

3. **The RN reports to the charge nurse that when she entered a client's room, the client threatened to cut herself with an unscrewed light bulb. Which priority intervention should the charge nurse plan to implement?**
   A. Call in an extra nurse or UAP for the next shift
   B. Assign one of the current UAPs to sit with the client
   C. Move the client to another room with a roommate
   D. Administer a PRN dose of lorazepam (Ativan) as prescribed

HESI Test Question Approach		
Positive?	**YES**	**NO**
Key Words		
Rephrase		
Rule Out Choices		
A	B	C	D

4. A UAP is assisting with the care of eight clients on a postpartum unit. Which assignment should the nurse delegate to the UAP?

   A. Check fundal firmness and lochia for the clients who delivered vaginally
   B. Take vital signs every 15 min for a client with pre-eclampsia
   C. Provide breast-feeding instructions for a primigravida
   D. Assist with daily care activities for the clients on bed rest

HESI Test Question Approach			
Positive?		**YES**	**NO**
Key Words			
Rephrase			
Rule Out Choices			
A	**B**	**C**	**D**

Advanced Clinical Concepts

5. Which client is at the highest risk for respiratory complications?

   A. A 21-year-old client with dehydration and cerebral palsy who is dependent in daily activities
   B. A 60-year-old client who has had type 2 diabetes for 20 years and who was admitted with cellulitis
   C. An obese 30-year-old client with hypertension who is noncompliant with the medication regimen
   D. A 40-year-old client, who takes a loop diuretic, who has a serum K^+ of 3.4 mmol/L (mEq/L) and complains of fatigue

HESI Test Question Approach			
Positive?		**YES**	**NO**
Key Words			
Rephrase			
Rule Out Choices			
A	**B**	**C**	**D**

6. A nurse stops at an accident and finds a young adult male lying next to an overturned truck. The victim is pulseless and apneic. What action has the highest priority?

   A. Initiate basic life support
   B. Remove the victim's clothing
   C. Assess for hemorrhage
   D. Remove glass shards from the victim's face

HESI Test Question Approach			
Positive?		**YES**	**NO**
Key Words			
Rephrase			
Rule Out Choices			
A	**B**	**C**	**D**

7. A client who is immediately postoperative for AAA repair has received normal saline intravenously at 125 mL/hr. The nurse observes dark yellow urine. The hourly output for the past 3 hours was 50 mL, 32 mL, and 28 mL. What action should the nurse take?

   A. Administer a bolus D_5 ½ NS at 200 mL/hr
   B. Contact the healthcare provider
   C. Monitor output for another 2 hours
   D. Draw blood samples for BUN and creatinine labs

HESI Test Question Approach		
Positive?	**YES**	**NO**
Key Words		
Rephrase		
Rule Out Choices		
A	B	C	D

8. The RN is evaluating the effects of administration of fresh frozen plasma (FFP) on a client in shock. Which finding(s) would indicate a positive outcome? (Select all that apply.)

   A. BUN–3.9 mmol/L (11 mg/dL); creatinine–62 mcmol/L (0.7mg/dL)
   B. Hemoglobin level of 100 mmol/L (10 gm/dL)
   C. Return of temperature to normal
   D. Decreased bleeding from the gums
   E. Negative guaiac for occult bleeding

HESI Test Question Approach		
Positive?	**YES**	**NO**
Key Words		
Rephrase		
Rule Out Choices		
A	B	C	D

9. A client's arterial blood gas results are: pH–7.29, pCO_2–55 mmHg, and HCO_3–26 mEq/L. Which compensatory response should the nurse expect to see?

   A. Respiratory rate of 30 breaths/min
   B. Apical rate of 120 beats/min
   C. Potassium level of 5.8 mmol/L (mEq/L)
   D. Complaints of pounding headache

HESI Test Question Approach		
Positive?	**YES**	**NO**
Key Words		
Rephrase		
Rule Out Choices		
A	B	C	D

10. A client with chronic back pain is not receiving adequate pain relief from oral analgesics. What alternative action should the nurse explore to promote the client's independence?
    A. Ask the healthcare provider to increase the analgesic dosage
    B. Obtain a prescription for a second analgesic, to be given by the IV route
    C. Consider the client's receptivity to complementary therapy
    D. Encourage counseling to prevent future addiction

HESI Test Question Approach			
Positive?		**YES**	**NO**
Key Words			
Rephrase			
Rule Out Choices			
A	B	C	D

| Maternal/Newborn Nursing

11. A client at 41 weeks' gestation who is in active labor calls the nurse to report that her membranes have ruptured. The nurse performs a vaginal examination and discovers that the umbilical cord has prolapsed. Which intervention should the nurse implement first?
    A. Elevate the presenting fetal part off the cord
    B. Cover the cord with sterile moist NS gauze
    C. Prepare for an emergency cesarean birth
    D. Administer O_2 by facemask at 10 L/min

HESI Test Question Approach			
Positive?		**YES**	**NO**
Key Words			
Rephrase			
Rule Out Choices			
A	B	C	D

12. A client at 39-weeks' gestation plans to have an epidural block when labor is established. What intervention(s) should the nurse implement to prevent side effects? (Select all that apply.)
    A. Teach the client about the procedure and effects of the epidural
    B. Place the client in a chair next to the bed
    C. Administer a bolus of 500 mL of normal saline solution
    D. Monitor the fetal heart rate and contractions continuously
    E. Assist the client to empty her bladder every two hours

HESI Test Question Approach			
Positive?		**YES**	**NO**
Key Words			
Rephrase			
Rule Out Choices			
A	B	C	D

13. A female client presents in the emergency department with RLQ abdominal pain and pain in her right shoulder. She has no vaginal bleeding, and her last menses was 6 weeks ago. Which actions should the nurse take first?
    A. Assess for abdominal rebound pain, distention, and fever
    B. Obtain VS, IV access, and notify the healthcare provider
    C. Observe for recent musculoskeletal injury, bruising, or abuse
    D. Collect specimens for pregnancy test, hemoglobin, and WBC count

HESI Test Question Approach			
Positive?		YES	NO
Key Words			
Rephrase			
Rule Out Choices			
A	B	C	D

14. A nurse has been assigned a pregnant client who has heart disease. The client's condition has been diagnosed as New York Heart Association (NYHA) Class II cardiac disease. What important fact(s) about activities of daily living while pregnant should the nurse teach this client? (Select all that apply.)
    A. Increase fiber in the diet
    B. Anticipate the need for rest breaks after physical activity
    C. Notify the healthcare provider if her rings do not fit
    D. Maintain bed rest with bathroom privileges
    E. Start a low-impact aerobic program

HESI Test Question Approach			
Positive?		YES	NO
Key Words			
Rephrase			
Rule Out Choices			
A	B	C	D

Medical-Surgical: Renal

15. A client is returning to the unit after an intravenous pyelogram (IVP). Which intervention should the nurse include in the client's plan of care?
    A. Maintain bed rest
    B. Increase fluid intake
    C. Monitor for hematuria
    D. Continue NPO status

HESI Test Question Approach			
Positive?		YES	NO
Key Words			
Rephrase			
Rule Out Choices			
A	B	C	D

16. The nurse is teaching a client who has chronic urinary tract infections about a prescription for ciprofloxacin (Cipro) 500mg PO bid. What side effect(s) could the client expect while taking this medication? (Select all that apply.)
    A. Photosensitivity
    B. Dyspepsia
    C. Diarrhea
    D. Urinary frequency
    E. Pernicious anemia

HESI Test Question Approach			
Positive?		YES	NO
Key Words			
Rephrase			
Rule Out Choices			
A	B	C	D

17. Which client complaint of pain requires the nurse's immediate intervention?
    A. Bladder pain while receiving a continuous saline irrigant 2 hours after a transurethral prostatic resection
    B. Incisional pain on postoperative day 3 after a nephrectomy; the client requests a PRN oral pain medication
    C. Flank pain that is partially relieved when the client passes a renal calculus
    D. Bladder spasms after draining 1,000 mL of urine during insertion of an indwelling catheter

HESI Test Question Approach			
Positive?		YES	NO
Key Words			
Rephrase			
Rule Out Choices			
A	B	C	D

18. A male client with a Tenckhoff catheter calls to report that he feels poorly and has a fever. What is the best response by the clinic nurse?
    A. Encourage him to come to the clinic today for assessment
    B. Instruct him to increase his fluid intake to 3 L/day
    C. Review his medication regimen for adherence
    D. Inquire about his recent dietary intake of protein and iron

HESI Test Question Approach			
Positive?		YES	NO
Key Words			
Rephrase			
Rule Out Choices			
A	B	C	D

19. The nurse is reviewing the cardiac markers for a client who was admitted immediately after reporting chest pain. Elevation of which laboratory value is the earliest marker for myocardial injury?
    A. Troponin levels
    B. Myoglobin level
    C. CK-MB level
    D. LDH level

HESI Test Question Approach			
Positive?		YES	NO
Key Words			
Rephrase			
Rule Out Choices			
A	B	C	D

20. The nurse is providing discharge instructions to a client who has been diagnosed with angina pectoris. Which instruction is most important?
    A. Avoid activity that involves the Valsalva maneuver
    B. Seek emergency treatment if chest pain persists after the third nitroglycerin dose
    C. Rest for 30 minutes after having chest pain before resuming activity
    D. Keep extra nitroglycerin in an airtight, light-resistant bottle

HESI Test Question Approach			
Positive?		YES	NO
Key Words			
Rephrase			
Rule Out Choices			
A	B	C	D

21. The nurse is providing discharge teaching for a client who has been prescribed diltiazem (Cardizem). Which dietary instruction has the highest priority?
    A. Maintain a low-sodium diet
    B. Eat a banana each morning
    C. Ingest high-fiber foods daily
    D. Avoid grapefruit products

HESI Test Question Approach			
Positive?		YES	NO
Key Words			
Rephrase			
Rule Out Choices			
A	B	C	D

22. The nurse is teaching a young adult female who has a history of Raynaud's disease how to control her pain. What information should the nurse offer?
    A. Take oral analgesics at regularly spaced intervals
    B. Avoid extremes of heat and cold
    C. Limit foods and fluids that contain caffeine
    D. Keep the affected extremities in a dependent position

HESI Test Question Approach			
Positive?		YES	NO
Key Words			
Rephrase			
Rule Out Choices			
A	B	C	D

23. The clinic nurse is caring for a client taking warfarin (Coumadin) for atrial fibrillation. Which client need should the nurse give highest priority?
    A. Having protamine sulfate available
    B. Teaching the client the importance of walking 10,000 steps daily
    C. Encouraging the client to eat brussels sprouts and cabbage
    D. Monitoring the platelet count for indications of thrombocytopenia

HESI Test Question Approach			
Positive?		YES	NO
Key Words			
Rephrase			
Rule Out Choices			
A	B	C	D

Medical-Surgical: Respiratory

24. A client who was admitted to the hospital with cancer of the larynx is scheduled for a laryngectomy tomorrow. What is the client's priority learning need tonight?
    A. Body image counseling
    B. Pain management expectations
    C. Communication techniques
    D. Postoperative nutritional needs

HESI Test Question Approach			
Positive?		YES	NO
Key Words			
Rephrase			
Rule Out Choices			
A	B	C	D

25. A victim of a motor vehicle collision is dead on arrival at the emergency department. What action should the nurse take to assist the spouse with this crisis?
    - A. Ask whether there is family, friends, or clergy to call
    - B. Talk about the former relationship with the spouse
    - C. Provide education about the stages of grief and loss
    - D. Assess the spouse's level of anxiety

HESI Test Question Approach			
Positive?		YES	NO
Key Words			
Rephrase			
Rule Out Choices			
A	B	C	D

26. The nurse is planning to lead a seminar for community health nurses on violence against women during pregnancy. Which statement describes an appropriate technique for assessing for violence?
    - A. Women should be assessed only if they are part of a high-risk group
    - B. Women may be assessed in the presence of young children, but not intimate partners
    - C. Women should be assessed once during pregnancy
    - D. Women should be reassessed face to face by a nurse as the pregnancy progresses

HESI Test Question Approach			
Positive?		YES	NO
Key Words			
Rephrase			
Rule Out Choices			
A	B	C	D

27. The charge nurse reminds clients on the mental health unit that breakfast is at 8 AM, medications are given at 9 AM, and group therapy sessions begin at 10 AM. Which treatment modality has been implemented?
    - A. Milieu therapy
    - B. Behavior modification
    - C. Peer therapy
    - D. Problem solving

HESI Test Question Approach			
Positive?		YES	NO
Key Words			
Rephrase			
Rule Out Choices			
A	B	C	D

28. The nurse is accompanying a client to the radiography department when he becomes panic stricken at the elevator and states, "I can't get on that elevator." Which action should the nurse take first?
    A. Ask one more staff member to ride in the elevator
    B. Offer a prescribed antianxiety medication
    C. Begin desensitization about riding the elevator
    D. Affirm the client's fears about riding the elevator

HESI Test Question Approach			
Positive?		YES	NO
Key Words			
Rephrase			
Rule Out Choices			
A	B	C	D

29. A client who experiences frequent nightmares and somnambulism is found one night trying to strangle his roommate. Which intervention is the nurse's highest priority?
    A. Give the client a sedative or hypnotic
    B. Administer an antipsychotic medication
    C. Move the client to a different room
    D. Process with both clients about the event

HESI Test Question Approach			
Positive?		YES	NO
Key Words			
Rephrase			
Rule Out Choices			
A	B	C	D

30. The nurse is updating the plan of care for a client who has a borderline personality disorder. Which intervention is most important to implement?
    A. Always assign the same nurse to care for the client
    B. Avoid challenging inappropriate behavior
    C. Limit the client's contact with other clients
    D. Remove consequences for acting-out behaviors

HESI Test Question Approach			
Positive?		YES	NO
Key Words			
Rephrase			
Rule Out Choices			
A	B	C	D

31. A female adolescent is admitted to the mental health unit for anorexia nervosa. In planning care, what is the nurse's highest priority?
    A. Teach the client the importance of self-expression
    B. Supervise the client's activities during the day
    C. Include the client in daily group therapy
    D. Facilitate social interactions with others

HESI Test Question Approach

Positive?		YES	NO
Key Words			
Rephrase			
Rule Out Choices			

A	B	C	D

32. The charge nurse is planning the daily schedule for clients on the mental health unit. A male client who is manic should be assigned to which activity?
    A. A basketball game in the gym
    B. Jogging at least 1 mile
    C. A ping-pong game with a peer
    D. Group therapy with the art therapist

HESI Test Question Approach

Positive?		YES	NO
Key Words			
Rephrase			
Rule Out Choices			

A	B	C	D

Leadership and Delegation

33. A nurse is planning the client assignments for the night shift. The nursing team includes a registered nurse, a licensed practical nurse, and two unlicensed assistive personnel (UAP). Which duty (or duties) could be delegated to the UAPs? (Select all that apply.)
    A. Transport a client who has had a stroke to the radiology department for a CAT scan
    B. Retrieve a unit of packed cells from the blood bank for a transfusion
    C. Bathe a 25-year-old client with sickle cell disease who has multiple IV lines and a PCA pump
    D. Turn a 92-year-old client who has end-stage heart failure and a DNR
    E. Page the HCP for a client with a fingerstick blood glucose level of 2.72 mmol/L (49 mg/dL)

HESI Test Question Approach

Positive?		YES	NO
Key Words			
Rephrase			
Rule Out Choices			

A	B	C	D

34. **A hospitalized client has been newly diagnosed with type 2 diabetes. Which task(s) can the RN delegate to the UAP? (Select all that apply.)**
    A. Contacting the dietitian for a prescribed consult
    B. Reporting the client's insulin injection technique
    C. Obtaining the fingerstick blood glucose level every ac and hs
    D. Reminding the client to dry the toes carefully after a shower
    E. Talking to the client about foods that raise the blood glucose level

HESI Test Question Approach			
Positive?		**YES**	**NO**
Key Words			
Rephrase			
Rule Out Choices			
A	B	C	D

35. **The home health nurse evaluates the insulin preparation and administration technique of a 36-year-old male client newly diagnosed with diabetes. The client has been prescribed insulin: lispro (Humalog) pen 10 units subcutaneously ac and Lantus 45 units subcutaneously once daily in AM. Which finding indicates that the client needs further education?**
    A. He mixes Lantus and lispro in the same syringe for the AM dose
    B. He leaves the insulin syringe in place for 5 seconds after injection
    C. He stores the opened insulin vials at room temperature in the cabinet
    D. He recaps and disposes of the single-use insulin syringe

HESI Test Question Approach			
Positive?		**YES**	**NO**
Key Words			
Rephrase			
Rule Out Choices			
A	B	C	D

36. **At change of shift, the charge nurse assigns the UAP four clients. The RN should direct the UAP to take vitals sign on which client first?**
    A. The 89-year-old with COPD who is resting quietly on 2 L of oxygen and who needs assistance with a bath
    B. The client who returned from endoscopy about 30 minutes ago and who is requesting something to eat
    C. The client newly diagnosed with type 2 diabetes who had a fingerstick glucose level of 4.2 mmol/L (75 mg/dL) and who needs help with breakfast
    D. The newly admitted client with rheumatoid arthritis who needs hand splints reapplied to both hands

HESI Test Question Approach			
Positive?		**YES**	**NO**
Key Words			
Rephrase			
Rule Out Choices			
A	B	C	D

37. After change of shift report, the nurse reviews her assignments. Which client should the nurse assess first?
   A. The elderly client receiving palliative care for heart failure who complains of constipation and nervousness
   B. The adult client who is 48 hours postoperative from a colectomy and who is reported to be having nausea
   C. The middle-aged client with chronic renal failure who has a urinary catheter that has been draining 95 mL for 8 hours
   D. The client who is 2 days postoperative from a thoracotomy and who has chest tubes, is on oxygen at 3 L/min, and has a respiratory rate of 12 breaths/min

HESI Test Question Approach			
Positive?		YES	NO
Key Words			
Rephrase			
Rule Out Choices			
A	B	C	D

38. The nurse is reviewing the laboratory values of her assigned clients. Which client has an abnormal lab report that the nurse should communicate immediately to the healthcare provider?
   A. The client who is post splenectomy after a motor vehicle accident and has a hemoglobin of 109 mmol/L (10.9 g/dL)
   B. The client receiving Coumadin (warfarin) who has an international normalized ratio (INR) of 2.3
   C. The 38-year-old client who is 24 hours post thyroidectomy and has a total calcium level of 2.35 mmol/L (9.4 mg/dL)
   D. The newly admitted client with a BUN of 10.7 mmol/L (30 mg/dL) and a creatinine of 97 mcmol/L (1.1 mg/dL)

HESI Test Question Approach			
Positive?		YES	NO
Key Words			
Rephrase			
Rule Out Choices			
A	B	C	D

39. The nurse receives a change of shift report on her four acute care clients. Which action should the nurse take first?
   A. Contact the healthcare provider for a prescription for an antiemetic on a postoperative client who has been vomiting
   B. Notify a family member of a client's impending transfer to Intensive Care Unit for angina and ST segment changes
   C. Inform the healthcare provider of a potassium level of 5.2 mmol/L (mEq/L) in the client with end-stage renal disease
   D. Begin assessment rounds, starting with the palliative care client having a diagnosis of heart failure

HESI Test Question Approach			
Positive?		YES	NO
Key Words			
Rephrase			
Rule Out Choices			
A	B	C	D

40. **The emergency department staff nurse is assigned four clients. Which client should the nurse assess first?**
    A. A preschooler with a barking cough, an O$_2$ sat of 93% on room air, and occasional inspiratory stridor
    B. A 10-month-old infant with a tympanic temperature of 38.9° C (102° F) and green nasal drainage who is pulling at her ears
    C. A crying 8-month-old with a harsh, paroxysmal cough; an audible expiratory wheeze; and mild retractions
    (D.) A clingy 3-year-old who has a sore throat and drooling and whose tongue is slightly protruding from his mouth

HESI Test Question Approach			
Positive?		YES	NO
Key Words			
Rephrase			
Rule Out Choices			
A	B	C	D

41. **The outpatient clinic nurse is reviewing phone messages from last night. Which client should the nurse call back first?**
    (A.) A woman at 30 weeks' gestation who has been diagnosed with mild pre-eclampsia; she was unable to relieve her heartburn
    B. A woman at 24 weeks' gestation who was crying about painful vulvar lesions and urinary frequency for the past 8 hours
    C. A woman at 12 weeks' gestation who was recently discharged from the hospital with hyperemesis gravidarum; she had had two episodes of vomiting in 6 hours
    D. A woman with type 1 diabetes who tested positive with a home pregnancy kit; she was worried about managing her diabetes

HESI Test Question Approach			
Positive?		YES	NO
Key Words			
Rephrase			
Rule Out Choices			
A	B	C	D

42. **The clinic nurse suspects that a 2-year-old child is being abused. What assessment finding(s) would support this? (Select all that apply.)**
    A. Petechiae in a straight line on the chest
    B. Gray-blue pigmented areas on the sacral region
    C. Bald patches on the scalp
    D. Ear tugging and crying
    E. Symmetrical burns on the hands

HESI Test Question Approach			
Positive?		YES	NO
Key Words			
Rephrase			
Rule Out Choices			
A	B	C	D

43. The nurse is caring for a client who had a thoracotomy 48 hours ago and now has left lower lobe chest tubes. The nurse notes that a chest tube is not tidaling. Which action should the nurse take first?
   A. Check for kinks in the chest drainage system
   B. Assess the heart rate and blood pressure
   C. Notify the rapid response team immediately
   D. Momentarily disconnect from wall suction

HESI Test Question Approach			
Positive?		YES	NO
Key Words			
Rephrase			
Rule Out Choices			
A	B	C	D

44. While the nurse is caring for a client who has had an MI, the monitor alarm sounds and the nurse notes ventricular fibrillation. What should be the nurse's first course of action?
   A. Notify the healthcare provider
   B. Increase the oxygen concentration
   C. Assess the client's level of consciousness
   D. Prepare to defibrillate the client

HESI Test Question Approach			
Positive?		YES	NO
Key Words			
Rephrase			
Rule Out Choices			
A	B	C	D

45. The physician has prescribed the removal of a client's internal jugular central line catheter. To remove the catheter safely, the nurse should give which intervention(s) the highest priority? (Select all that apply.)
   A. Carefully remove the Bioderm dressing
   B. Place the client in the Trendelenburg position
   C. Send the catheter tip to the lab for a C & S
   D. Have the client take a deep breath during removal
   E. Apply pressure for 20 minutes after removal of the catheter

HESI Test Question Approach			
Positive?		YES	NO
Key Words			
Rephrase			
Rule Out Choices			
A	B	C	D

Answers and Rationales

(Correct answers are underlined.)

Management/Leadership

1. **Which activity should the nurse delegate to an unlicensed assistive personnel (UAP)?**

Rationales:

A. *Check to see whether a client with cirrhosis can hear any better today after discontinuation of an IV antibiotic*
This requires assessment about ototoxicity, which is beyond the scope of practice of a UAP.

B. *Encourage additional PO fluids for an elderly client with pneumonia who has developed a fever*
These directions are not sufficiently clear and detailed for the UAP to perform the task.

C. *Report the ability of a client with myasthenia gravis to manage the supper tray independently*
This requires assessment of the client's clinical status, which is beyond the scope of the UAP.

D. <u>*Record the number of liquid stools of a client who received lactulose for an elevated NH_3 level*</u>
This task encompasses basic care, elimination, and intake and output; it does not require judgment or the expertise of the nurse and can be performed by the UAP.

2. **The nurse is assigning clients to the UAP. Which client requires intervention by the RN?**

Rationales:

A. *The client with active TB who is leaving the room without a mask*
A UAP can be delegated to provide a box of masks or to direct the client back to the room.

B. *The client with dehydration who is requesting something to drink*
A UAP can be directed to provide specific types and amounts of fluids.

C. <u>*The client with asthma who complains of being anxious and cannot concentrate*</u>
This client requires assessment and is at risk for airway compromise, which also requires assessment, so the nurse should attend to this client.

D. *The client with COPD who is leaving the unit to smoke, even though the next IVPB is due*
A UAP can ask the client to delay leaving the unit.

3. **The RN reports to the charge nurse that when she entered a client's room, the client threatened to cut herself with an unscrewed light bulb. Which priority intervention should the charge nurse plan to implement?**

Rationales:

A. *Call in an extra nurse or UAP for the next shift*
The charge nurse should plan ahead for staffing, but the immediate focus should be the client's safety now.

B. <u>*Assign one of the current UAPs to sit with the client*</u>
Because the client is at risk for suicide, the charge nurse should assign a staff member to stay with the client.

C. *Move the client to another room with a roommate*
This will not ensure the client's safety; also, a staff member, not another client, must be present with the client at all times.

D. *Administer a PRN dose of lorazepam (Ativan) as prescribed*
Although the client may be anxious, this is not a priority intervention that would ensure her safety.

4. **A UAP is assisting with the care of eight clients on a postpartum unit. Which assignment should the nurse delegate to the UAP?**

Rationales:

A. *Check fundal firmness and lochia for the clients who delivered vaginally*
Assessment is a responsibility of the nurse.

B. *Take vital signs every 15 minutes for a client with pre-eclampsia*
This is a high-risk patient who needs to be evaluated by a licensed nurse.

C. *Provide breast-feeding instructions for a primigravida*
Teaching is also the responsibility of the RN.

D. <u>*Assist with daily care activities for the clients on bed rest*</u>
This is the most appropriate assignment for the UAP. The RN should delegate daily care activities to the UAP based on the RN's assessments of each client's needs.

Advanced Clinical Concepts

5. **Which client is at the highest risk for respiratory complications?**

Rationales:

A. <u>*A 21-year-old client with dehydration and cerebral palsy who is dependent in daily activities*</u>
A client with dehydration and cerebral palsy (characterized by uncoordinated, spastic muscle movements) that affects ADL independence is at increased risk for respiratory problems because of impaired mobility and impaired swallowing.

B. *A 60-year-old client who has had type 2 diabetes for 20 years who was admitted with cellulitis*
This older client is more at risk for renal, cardiac, and vascular complications.

C. *An obese 30-year-old client with hypertension who is noncompliant with the medication regimen*
An obese adult who is noncompliant with antihypertensive medications is more at risk for cardiac or cerebral events than for respiratory problems.

D. *A 40-year-old client, who takes a loop diuretic, who has a serum K^+ of 3.4 mmol/L (mEq/L) and complains of fatigue*
This middle-aged adult is hypokalemic and fatigued but is not at high risk for respiratory problems.

6. **A nurse stops at an accident and finds a young adult male lying next to an overturned truck. The victim is pulseless and apneic. What action has the highest priority?**

Rationales:

A. ***Initiate basic life support***

Initiating CPR is vital to this victim's survival and is the first priority.

B. *Remove the victim's clothing*

The victim's clothing should be removed so that he can be examined for any underlying signs of illness or injury; however, this is not the priority.

C. *Assess for hemorrhage*

Accident victims are at risk for internal or external hemorrhage; however, this assessment does not have the highest priority.

D. *Remove glass shards from the victim's face*

Other life-threatening situations require action before the removal of glass.

7. **A client who is immediately postoperative for AAA repair has received normal saline intravenously at 125 mL/hr. The nurse observes dark yellow urine. The hourly output for the past 3 hours was 50 mL, 32 mL, and 28 mL. What action should the nurse take?**

Rationales:

A. *Administer a bolus D_5 ½ NS at 200 mL/hr*

This action is not recommended, because hypertonic solutions are prescribed for fluid and electrolyte imbalances and cause an osmotic movement of fluids into the vasculature.

B. ***Contact the healthcare provider***

Low urinary output may be a serious problem and requires more immediate intervention from the HCP.

C. *Monitor output for another 2 hours*

Urine output has been monitored and may indicate dehydration, which can lead to more serious complications.

D. *Draw blood samples for BUN and creatinine labs*

The BUN and creatinine should be evaluated, but that is not the immediate priority.

8. **The RN is evaluating the effects of administration of fresh frozen plasma (FFP) on a client in shock. Which finding(s) would indicate a positive outcome? (Select all that apply.)**

Rationales:

A. *BUN–3.9 mmol/L (11 mg/dL); creatinine–62 mcmol/L (0.7mg/dL)*

BUN and creatinine levels are important to evaluate in a client in shock; however, these values are not affected by administration of FFP.

B. *Hemoglobin level of 100 mmol/L (10 gm/dL)*

FFP does not affect hemoglobin levels.

C. *Return of temperature to normal*

Although monitoring the client's temperature is important, FFP does not have a direct effect on this parameter.

D. ***Decreased bleeding from the gums***

FFP replaces clotting factors; therefore, detecting occult (hidden) bleeding and obvious bleeding provides valuable information.

E. ***Negative guaiac for occult bleeding***

Detecting occult (hidden) bleeding and obvious bleeding provides valuable information.

9. **A client's arterial blood gas results are pH–7.29, pCO_2–55 mmHg, and HCO_3–26 mEq/L. Which compensatory response should the nurse expect to see?**

Rationales:

A. *Respiratory rate of 30 breaths/min*

The client is experiencing respiratory acidosis. Tachypnea does not produce compensation in respiratory acidosis.

B. *Apical rate of 120 beats/min*

Acid-base imbalances are compensated primarily by the lungs and the renal system. Plasma proteins and ionic shifts (intracellular) also serve as buffering systems. Tachycardia, does not serve as a compensatory mechanism.

C. ***Potassium level of 5.8 mmol/L (mEq/L)***

To compensate for the acidosis created by increased CO_2, K^+ ions are released from cellular proteins and H^+ ions take their place, bound to the proteins. The result is frequently serum hyperkalemia.

D. *Complaints of a pounding headache*

Headache may be a manifestation of CO_2 retention, but it is not a compensatory mechanism for respiratory acidosis.

10. **A client with chronic back pain is not receiving adequate pain relief from oral analgesics. What alternative action should the nurse explore to promote the client's independence?**

Rationales:

A. *Ask the healthcare provider to increase the analgesic dosage*

Although this intervention may improve pain relief, it may not promote self-care without increasing side effects that could affect the client's independence.

B. *Obtain a prescription for a second analgesic, to be given by the IV route*

The IV route does not promote self-care and may cause additional side effects that interfere with the client's ability to carry out ADLs independently.

C. ***Consider the client's receptivity to complementary therapy***

This action supports self-care without the high level of adverse effects associated with additional medication.

It is the least invasive measure, and it promotes the active participation (self-care) of the client.

D. **Encourage counseling to prevent future addiction**
Referrals may be needed, but the nurse should teach clients about potential problems with medications and measures to manage pain and maintain self-care.

Maternal-Newborn Nursing

11. **A client at 41 weeks' gestation who is in active labor calls the nurse to report that her membranes have ruptured. The nurse performs a vaginal examination and discovers that the umbilical cord has prolapsed. Which intervention should the nurse implement first?**

Rationales:

A. <u>*Elevate the presenting fetal part off the cord*</u>
This action is the most critical intervention. The nurse must prevent compression of the cord by the presenting part, because that would impair fetal circulation, leading to both morbidity and death.

B. **Cover the cord with sterile moist NS gauze**
If the cord is protruding outside the vagina, this action should be taken to prevent drying of the Wharton's jelly. However, another nurse should do this while the first nurse maintains elevation of the presenting part off the cord.

C. **Prepare for an emergency cesarean birth**
This is implemented by the staff while the nurse keeps the presenting part elevated off the cord.

D. **Administer O₂ by facemask at 10 L/min**
Oxygen should be provided to the mother to increase oxygen delivery to the fetus via the placenta; however, another nurse should do this while first the nurse keeps the presenting part elevated off the cord.

12. **A client at 39-weeks' gestation plans to have an epidural block when labor is established. What intervention(s) should the nurse implement to prevent side effects? (Select all that apply.)**

Rationales:

A. **Teach the client about the procedure and effects of the epidural**
Teaching is an important nursing intervention to alleviate anxiety, but it does not prevent hypotension, a side effect due to vasodilation caused by the epidural block.

B. **Place the client in a chair next to the bed**
Epidural block reduces lower extremity sensation and movement to varying degrees. Any upright positions such as walking and standing may not be possible during epidural pain management and may not prevent side effects.

C. <u>*Administer a bolus of 500 mL of normal saline solution*</u>
Prehydration increases maternal blood volume and prevents hypotension, which occurs as a result of

vasodilation, a side effect of epidural anesthesia. A saline solution is used to prevent fetal secretion of insulin that later places the neonate at risk for hypoglycemia.

D. <u>*Monitor the fetal heart rate and contractions continuously*</u>
Vital signs should be monitored every 5 minutes immediately after the initial epidural dose, and if the client's condition is stable, then every 15 minutes.

E. <u>*Assist the client to empty her bladder every 2 hours*</u>
Assisting the client to void every 2 hours prevents bladder distention.

13. **A female client presents in the emergency department with RLQ abdominal pain and pain in her right shoulder. She has no vaginal bleeding, and her last menses was 6 weeks ago. Which actions should the nurse take first?**

Rationales:

A. **Assess for abdominal rebound pain, distention, and fever**
Bleeding related to an ectopic pregnancy (based on the client's history) may present these manifestations, but the nurse should first assess the client for hypovolemic shock.

B. <u>*Obtain VS, IV access, and notify the healthcare provider*</u>
The nurse should first evaluate the client for vital sign changes of shock due to a ruptured ectopic pregnancy (an obstetrical emergency). A vascular access is vital in an emergency situation, and the healthcare provider should be notified immediately.

C. **Observe for recent musculoskeletal injury, bruising, or abuse**
This may be part of the assessment if a life-threatening situation is ruled out first.

D. **Collect specimens for pregnancy test, hemoglobin, and WBC count**
Specimens for a pregnancy test and CBC should be collected. However, the nurse should first notify the healthcare provider of the client's status, based on the presenting vital signs and symptoms of bleeding, as manifested by intraabdominal bleeding that collects under the diaphragm, causing referred shoulder pain.

14. **A nurse has been assigned a pregnant client who has heart disease. The client's condition has been diagnosed as New York Heart Association (NYHA) Class II cardiac disease. What important fact(s) about activities of daily living while pregnant should the nurse teach this client? (Select all that apply.)**

Rationales:

A. <u>*Increase fiber in the diet*</u>
ADL restrictions for clients with NYHA Class II cardiac disease create a risk factor for constipation.

177

B. Anticipate the need for rest breaks after physical activity

Individuals with NYHA Class II cardiac disease may have limitations on activity.

C. Notify the healthcare provider if her rings do not fit anymore

Tight rings may indicate weight gain, and the client may be at risk for CHF.

D. Maintain bed rest with bathroom privileges

It is not necessary to maintain bed rest for a client with NYHA Class II cardiac disease.

E. Start a low-impact aerobic program

Individuals with NYHA Class II cardiac disease may have some slight limitation of activity. During pregnancy, women may progress from Class I or II to Class III or IV as cardiac output increases and more stress is placed on the heart.

Medical-Surgical: Renal

15. A client is returning to the unit after an intravenous pyelogram (IVP). Which intervention should the nurse include in the client's plan of care?

Rationales:

A. Maintain bed rest

There is no need to restrict mobility after an IVP.

B. Increase fluid intake

The client should increase the fluid intake to clear the dye used in an IVP, because the dye may damage the kidneys.

C. Monitor for hematuria

There is no risk of hematuria related to an IVP.

D. Continue NPO status

The client does not need to be NPO after an IVP. Fluids should be increased.

16. The nurse is teaching a client who has chronic urinary tract infections about a prescription for ciprofloxacin (Cipro) 500 mg PO bid. What side effect(s) could the client expect while taking this medication? (Select all that apply.)

Rationales:

A. Photosensitivity

This is a side effect of Cipro; exposure to sunlight or tanning beds should be avoided. The client should be instructed to use sunscreen and protective clothing.

B. Dyspepsia

Cipro causes GI irritation, nausea and vomiting, and abdominal pain, which should be reported.

C. Diarrhea

Watery, foul-smelling diarrhea is an adverse reaction to Cipro that indicates pseudomembranous colitis; this should be reported and requires immediate intervention.

D. Urinary frequency

Urinary frequency may indicate that the medication is ineffective and should be reported.

E. Pernicious anemia

This is not a side effect of Cipro.

17. Which client complaint of pain requires the nurse's immediate intervention?

Rationales:

A. Bladder pain while receiving a continuous saline irrigant 2 hours after a transurethral prostatic resection

This client is at risk of clot formation occluding the catheter, and the pain may indicate bleeding and bladder distention; the nurse should evaluate this client immediately.

B. Incisional pain on postoperative day 3 after a nephrectomy; the client requests a PRN oral pain medication

This is not as high a priority compared to option A, because the client is not at risk of altered homeostasis.

C. Flank pain that is partially relieved when the client passes a renal calculus

This client's condition is not likely to worsen now that the stone was passed; it should be evaluated after the client in option A.

D. Bladder spasms after draining 1000 mL of urine during insertion of an indwelling catheter

This client's pain reflects the bladder spasms and is a lower priority than option A.

18. A male client with a Tenckhoff catheter calls to report he feels poorly and has a fever. What is the best response by the clinic nurse?

Rationales:

A. Encourage him to come to the clinic today for assessment

Tenckhoff catheters are used in peritoneal dialysis. They are often used at home by the client, placing the client at risk for peritoneal infection. Because dialysis clients usually have some degree of compromised immunity and anemia, the client should come to the clinic for assessment.

B. Instruct him to increase his fluid intake to 3 L/day

Clients who need dialysis retain fluid and usually are restricted to an intake that is only 300 mL greater than output.

C. Review his medication regimen for adherence

The nurse should evaluate the client's adherence, but assessing him for infection is a higher priority.

D. Inquire about his recent dietary intake of protein and iron

Iron deficiency and protein loss are common problems in clients who are receiving peritoneal dialysis. Dietary intake is important, but it is not a higher priority than possible infection.

19. The nurse is reviewing the cardiac markers for a client who was admitted immediately after reporting chest pain. Elevation of which laboratory value is the earliest marker for myocardial injury?

Rationales:

A. Troponin levels
A rise in the troponin levels is diagnostic of myocardial injury. cTnT and cTnI are detectable within hours of myocardial injury (4 to 6 hours, on average); the levels peak at 10 to 24 hours and can be detected for up to 10 to 14 days.

B. <u>Myoglobin level</u>
Myoglobin is cleared from the circulation rapidly and is most diagnostic if measured within the first 12 hours after the onset of chest pain. Serum concentrations rise 30 to 60 minutes after an MI.

C. CK-MB level
This isoenzyme is useful for supporting a diagnosis of MI and in determining the extent and time of the infarct. This marker usually returns to normal in 72 hours and is less useful in the nonacute phase.

D. LDH level
The LDH level rises within 24 to 48 hours after myocardial injury and returns to normal in about 5 to 10 days. Isolated elevation of this isoenzyme is especially useful as a delayed indicator of myocardial injury.

20. The nurse is providing discharge instructions to a client who has been diagnosed with angina pectoris. Which instruction is most important?

Rationales:

A. Avoid activity that involves the Valsalva maneuver
Although minimizing or avoiding the Valsalva maneuver decreases anginal pain; this is not the most important factor.

B. <u>Seek emergency treatment if chest pain persists after the third nitroglycerin dose</u>
This instruction is most important, because chest pain characteristic of acute MI persists longer than 15 minutes, and delaying medical treatment can be life threatening.

C. Rest for 30 minutes after having chest pain before resuming activity
Waiting 30 minutes may be recommended only if the nitroglycerin is effective in relieving the chest pain.

D. Keep extra nitroglycerin in an airtight, light-resistant bottle
This is excellent medication teaching, but it does not have the same urgency as seeking emergency care.

21. The nurse is providing discharge teaching for a client who has been prescribed diltiazem (Cardizem). Which dietary instruction has the highest priority?

Rationales:

A. Maintain a low-sodium diet
The client may need to restrict sodium intake, but it is not specific for Cardizem.

B. Eat a banana each morning
If the client has low potassium, this should be recommended.

C. Ingest high-fiber foods daily
This is an excellent teaching point for everyone, but it is not specific for Cardizem.

D. <u>Avoid grapefruit products</u>
Grapefruit should be avoided during therapy with calcium channel blockers, because it can cause an increase in the serum drug level, predisposing the client to hypotension.

22. The nurse is teaching a young adult female who has a history of Raynaud's disease how to control her pain. What information should the nurse offer?

Rationales:

A. Take oral analgesics at regularly spaced intervals
Pain is not always associated with Raynaud's disease, as is the feeling of cold hands and fingers and pallor. If pain is sporadic or situational, it should not require regular use of analgesics.

B. <u>Avoid extremes of heat and cold</u>
In Raynaud's disease, vascular spasms of the hands and fingers are triggered by exposure to extremes of heat or cold, which causes the characteristic pallor and cold-to-the-touch symptoms of the upper extremities.

C. Limit food and fluids that contain caffeine
Caffeine is not the primary trigger of the episodes; however, if the client notes that caffeine contributes to the blanching and coldness, it should be avoided.

D. Keep the affected extremities in a dependent position
This is not effective for a client with Raynaud's disease.

23. The clinic nurse is caring for a client taking warfarin (Coumadin) for atrial fibrillation. Which client need should the nurse give highest priority?

Rationales:

A. Having protamine sulfate available
Protamine sulfate is the antidote for heparin.

B. Teaching the client the importance of walking 10,000 steps daily
Low-impact exercise, such as walking, is best for clients prescribed Coumadin; however, this is not the highest priority.

C. Encouraging the client to eat brussels sprouts and cabbage

Brussels sprouts and cabbage are foods high in vitamin K and would not be encouraged.

D. _Monitoring the platelet count for indications of thrombocytopenia_

Thrombocytopenia is a low platelet count. Platelets are essential for initiating the normal clotting mechanism. Coumadin therapy puts this client at risk for injury and bleeding.

Medical-Surgical: Respiratory

24. **A client who was admitted to the hospital with cancer of the larynx is scheduled for a laryngectomy tomorrow. What is the client's priority learning need tonight?**

Rationales:

A. Body image counseling

This is a concern after surgery, when the immediate life-threatening insult of cancer has been assimilated and basic needs have been met.

B. Pain management expectations

Pain relief expectations are a priority, but the inability to convey (communicate) a subjective symptom, such as pain, is the fear the client perceives first.

C. _Communication techniques_

A client who is in crisis and anticipating the immediate postoperative period is concerned with immediate needs, such as the ability to express and convey a subjective symptom (e.g., pain) and obtain intervention.

D. Postoperative nutritional needs

Nutrition is important to promote healing, but the ability to communicate subjective needs is a higher priority.

Psychiatric Nursing

25. **A victim of a motor vehicle collision is dead on arrival at the emergency department. What action should the nurse take to assist the spouse with this crisis?**

Rationales:

A. _Ask whether there is family, friends, or clergy to call_

The nurse should help the spouse identify support systems and resources that are helpful in coping with a crisis situation, such as the sudden death of a spouse.

B. Talk about the former relationship with the spouse

The spouse may be unable to process information during the crisis, and the nurse should focus on immediate needs for coping and support.

C. Provide education about the stages of grief and loss

Educating the client about grief and loss is not an immediate priority in a crisis and should be provided after the spouse begins to cope with the situation.

D. Assess the spouse's level of anxiety

Although the nurse should assess the spouse for anxiety, the immediate intervention should include a directive approach to assist the spouse in dealing with the stressful event.

26. **The nurse is planning to lead a seminar for community health nurses on violence against women during pregnancy. Which statement describes an appropriate technique for assessing for violence?**

Rationales:

A. Women should be assessed only if they are part of high-risk groups

Violence against women occurs in all ethnic groups and at all income levels.

B. Women may be assessed in the presence of young children but not intimate partners

It is important to assess women without their partners present; it is also important that verbal children not be present, because they may repeat what is heard. Infants may be present.

C. Women should be assessed once during pregnancy

Many women do not reveal violence the first time they are asked. As trust develops between the nurse and the client, the woman may be more comfortable sharing her story. Also, violence may start later in the pregnancy.

D. _Women should be reassessed face to face by a nurse as the pregnancy progresses_

More than one face-to-face interview elicits the highest reports of violence during pregnancy.

27. **The charge nurse reminds clients on the mental health unit that breakfast is at 8 AM, medications are given at 9 AM, and group therapy sessions begin at 10 AM. Which treatment modality has been implemented?**

Rationales:

A. _Milieu therapy_

Milieu therapy uses resources and activities in the environment to assist with improving social functioning and activities of daily living.

B. Behavior modification

Behavior modification involves changing behaviors using positive and negative reinforcements to allow desired activities or remove privileges.

C. Peer therapy

Peer therapy is not a single therapeutic modality; it involves the interaction of peers who are responsible for supporting, sharing, and compromising within their peer group and milieu.

D. Problem solving

Problem solving is used in crisis intervention; it focuses on problem identification and ways to return to previous levels of functioning.

28. The nurse is accompanying a client to the radiography department when he becomes panic stricken at the elevator and states, "I can't get on that elevator." Which action should the nurse take first?

Rationales:

A. *Ask one more staff member to ride the elevator*
One more staff member will not be able to mobilize the client to ride the elevator, because the client must first recognize his feelings about the phobia and accept the need to change his behavior.

B. *Offer a prescribed antianxiety medication*
Offering an antianxiety medication may be needed to proceed with desensitization.

C. *Begin desensitization about riding the elevator*
Desensitizing the client may be implemented, but first the client should identify his fears and recognize his anxiety.

D. *Affirm the client's fears about riding the elevator*
The nurse should first validate and allow the client to affirm his anxiety and fears about riding the elevator. Then options to initiate desensitization may be considered.

29. A client who experiences frequent nightmares and somnambulism is found one night trying to strangle his roommate. Which intervention is the nurse's highest priority?

Rationales:

A. *Give the client a sedative or hypnotic*
Sleepwalking is more likely to occur when a client is fatigued, anxious, and has received a hypnotic or sedative; safety is the priority.

B. *Administer an antipsychotic medication*
An antipsychotic medication is indicated if the client is psychotic and agitated; however, the nurse should ensure the safety of both clients first.

C. *Move the client to a different room*
The nurse should implement safety precautions immediately and move the client to a private room to protect both clients from harm or retaliation.

D. *Process with both clients about the event*
Although both clients should talk about the incident, this is not an opportune time, and the clients should be separated to provide a safe environment.

30. The nurse is updating the plan of care for a client who has a borderline personality disorder. Which intervention is most important to implement?

Rationales:

A. *Always assign the same nurse to care for the client*
The best intervention is to provide consistency and avoid splitting by assigning the client to only one nurse.

B. *Avoid challenging inappropriate behavior*
The nurse should assist the client to recognize manipulative behavior and set limits on manipulative behaviors as necessary.

C. *Limit the client's contact with other clients*
Socialization should be encouraged to improve the client's social skills.

D. *Remove consequences for acting-out behavior*
Firm limits with clear expectations and consequences are needed for manipulative clients.

31. A female adolescent is admitted to the mental health unit for anorexia nervosa. In planning care, what is the nurse's highest priority?

Rationales:

A. *Teach the client the importance of self-expression*
Self-expression of feelings is important, but re-establishing normal eating habits and physiological integrity is the priority intervention.

B. *Supervise the client's activities during the day*
The nurse should monitor and supervise the client's activities to prevent binging, purging, or avoiding meals.

C. *Include the client in daily group therapy*
The client should be included in daily groups, but the priority is physiological needs and monitoring meals.

D. *Facilitate social interactions with others*
The client should be given opportunities to socialize, but monitoring activities during the day, especially meals, is the priority.

32. The charge nurse is planning the daily schedule for clients on the mental health unit. A male client who is manic should be assigned to which activity?

Rationales:

A. *A basketball game in the gym*
The client should avoid any potentially competitive physical activity, especially contact sports, that can stimulate aggressive acting out.

B. *Jogging at least 1 mile*
Jogging is the best activity for this client, because it is a noncompetitive physical activity, and it requires the use of large muscle groups that expend energy associated with mania.

C. *A ping-pong game with a peer*
The client should not be assigned to any competitive activities that can frustrate him and stimulate mood swings.

D. *Group therapy with the art therapist*
A manic client may become disruptive and distracted in an art group; physical activity using large muscle groups is more effective in expending energy.

Leadership and Delegation

33. A nurse is planning the client assignments for the night shift. The nursing team includes a registered nurse, a licensed practical nurse and two unlicensed assistive personnel (UAP) on the nursing team. Which duties could be delegated to the UAPs? (Select all that apply.)

Rationales:
A. *Transport a client who has had a stroke to the radiology department for a CAT scan*
B. *Retrieve a unit of packed cells from the blood bank for a transfusion*
C. *Bathe a 25-year-old client with sickle cell disease who has multiple IV lines and a PCA pump*
D. *Turn a 92-year-old client who has end-stage heart failure and a DNR*
E. *Page the HCP for a client with a fingerstick blood glucose level of 49 mg/dL*

The UAP can perform noninvasive and nonsterile activities (options A, C, and D); collects and reports data such as vital signs, height and weight, and capillary blood glucose results; assist with socialization; and perform clerical duties (E).

34. A hospitalized client has been newly diagnosed with type 2 diabetes. Which task(s) can the RN delegate to the UAP? (Select all that apply.)

Rationales:
A. *Contacting the dietitian for a prescribed consult*
B. *Reporting the client's insulin injection technique*
C. *Obtaining the fingerstick blood glucose level every ac and hs*
D. *Reminding the client to dry the toes carefully after a shower*
E. *Talking to the client about foods that raise the blood glucose level*

The UAP can collect and report data such as vital signs, height and weight, and capillary blood sugar results (option C); perform hygiene tasks (option D); and carry out clerical duties (option A). Clients who need education or reinforcement of education require intervention by the RN or PN (options B and E).

35. The home health nurse evaluates the insulin preparation and administration technique of a 36-year-old male client newly diagnosed with diabetes. The client has been prescribed insulin: lispro (Humalog) pen 10 units subcutaneously ac and Lantus 45 units subcutaneously once daily in AM. Which finding indicates that the client needs further education?

Rationales:
A. *He mixes Lantus and lispro in the same syringe for the AM dose*
Lantus must not be mixed with any other insulin or dilutions.

B. *He leaves the insulin syringe in place for 5 seconds after injection.*
The pen must be held with the needle in place for 5 seconds to ensure that all insulin has been injected.
C. *He stores the opened insulin vials at room temperature in the cabinet.*
Insulin is stored at room temperature, out of direct sunlight.
D. *He recaps and disposes of the single-use insulin syringe.*
Clients may recap needles, but healthcare providers may not to reduce the risk of needlestick injury.

36. At change of shift, the charge nurse assigns the UAP four clients. The RN should direct the UAP to take vitals signs on which client first?

Rationales:
A. *The 89-year-old with COPD who is resting quietly on 2 L of oxygen and who needs assistance with a bath*
This client is stable.
B. *The client who returned from endoscopy about 30 minutes ago and who is requesting something to eat*
This client needs to have his vital signs taken to determine his stability after endoscopy; this is a priority.
C. *The client newly diagnosed with type 2 diabetes who had a fingerstick blood glucose level of 4.2 mmol/L (75 mg/dL) and who needs help with breakfast*
This client is stable.
D. *The newly admitted client with rheumatoid arthritis who needs to have hand splints reapplied to both hands*
This client is stable.

37. After change of shift report, the nurse reviews her assignments. Which client should the nurse assess first?

Rationales:
A. *The elderly client receiving palliative care for heart failure who complains of constipation and nervousness*
Constipation and nervousness are expected and common complications of palliative care.
B. *The adult client who is 48 hours postoperative from a colectomy and who is reported to be having nausea*
Nausea is the most common postoperative complication; it should be an assessment priority.
C. *The middle-aged client with chronic renal failure who has a urinary catheter that has been draining 95 mL for 8 hours*
Urine output varies, depending on the stage of chronic renal failure.

D. The client who is 2 days postoperative from a thoracotomy and who has chest tubes, is on oxygen at 3 L/min, and has a respiratory rate of 12 breaths/min

This respiratory rate is within normal limits.

38. **The nurse is reviewing the laboratory values of her assigned clients. Which client has an abnormal lab report that the nurse should communicate immediately to the healthcare provider?**

Rationales:

A. *The client who is post splenectomy after a motor vehicle accident and has a hemoglobin of 109 mmol/L (10.9 g/dL)*

This lab value may require action, but it is not the priority.

B. *The client receiving Coumadin (warfarin) who has a international normalized ratio (INR) of 2.3*

This lab value may require action, but it is not the priority.

C. *The 38-year-old client who is 24 hours post thyroidectomy and has a total calcium level of 2.35 mmol/L (9.4 mg/dL)*

This lab value may require action, but it is not the priority.

D. <u>*The newly admitted client who has a BUN of 10.7 mmol/L (30 mg/dL) and a creatinine of 97 mcmol/L (1.1 mg/dL)*</u>

The normal BUN-to-creatinine ratio is 10-20:1. A BUN that is disproportionally elevated raises suspicion of dehydration; the nurse should notify the HCP immediately.

39. **The nurse receives a change of shift report on her four acute care clients. Which action should the nurse take first?**

Rationales:

A. <u>*Contact the healthcare provider for a prescription for an antiemetic on a postoperative client who has been vomiting*</u>

Postoperative nausea and vomiting (PONV) are among the most common reactions after surgery. PONV can stress and irritate abdominal and GI wounds, increase intracranial pressure in patients who had head and neck surgery, elevate intraocular pressure in patients who had eye surgery, and increase the risk for aspiration. Obtaining a prescription for relieving PONV will decrease these risks.

B. *Notify a family member of a client's impending transfer to Intensive Care Unit for angina and ST segment changes.*

This is a change in status and should be performed after managing the PONV

C. *Inform the healthcare provider of a potassium level of 5.2 mmol/L (mEq/L) in the client with end-stage renal disease.*

This is an expected outcome of ESRD

D. *Begin assessment rounds, starting with the palliative care client having a diagnosis of heart failure.*

Assessing the client receiving palliative care is important however managing the client with PONV is the priority

40. **The emergency department staff nurse is assigned four clients. Which client should the nurse assess first?**

Rationales:

A. *A preschooler with a barking cough, an O_2 sat of 93% on room air, and occasional inspiratory stridor*

This is not a medical emergency but may require intervention.

B. *A 10-month-old with a tympanic temperature of 38.9° C (102° F) and green nasal drainage and who is pulling at her ears*

This is not a medical emergency but may require intervention.

C. *A crying 8-month-old with a harsh, paroxysmal cough; an audible expiratory wheeze; and mild retractions*

This is not a medical emergency but may require intervention.

D. <u>*A clingy 3-year-old who has a sore throat and drooling and whose tongue slightly protrudes from his mouth*</u>

Drooling, a history of sore throat, and a protruding tongue are classic manifestations of epiglottis; this is a medical emergency.

41. **The outpatient clinic nurse is reviewing phone messages from last night. Which client should the nurse call back first?**

Rationales:

A. <u>*A woman at 30 weeks' gestation who has been diagnosed with mild pre-eclampsia; she was unable to relieve her heartburn*</u>

A sign of a potential complication of eclampsia is epigastric pain, which may be indicative of liver damage and HELLP syndrome, a medical emergency.

B. *A woman at 24 weeks' gestation who was crying about painful vulvar lesions and urinary frequency for the past 8 hours*

This is a reasonable concern, but it does not take priority over option A.

C. *A woman at 12 weeks' gestation who was recently discharged from the hospital with hyperemesis gravidarum; she had had two episodes of vomiting in 6 hours*

This is a reasonable concern, but it does not take priority over option A.

D. *A woman with type 1 diabetes who tested positive with a home pregnancy kit; she was worried about managing her diabetes*

This is a reasonable concern, but it does not take priority over option A.

42. The clinic nurse suspects that a 2-year-old child is being abused. What assessment finding(s) would support this? (Select all that apply)

Rationales:

A. *Petechiae in a straight line on the chest*
Petechiae on the chest may be the result of the coining procedure, a cultural practice among Southeast Asian populations.

B. *Gray-blue pigmented areas on the sacral region*
These are Mongolian spots, blue areas commonly located on the sacral region that are consistent in shape and color.

C. *Bald patches on the scalp*
Bald patches typically are symmetrical and are indicative of physical abuse.

D. *Ear tugging and crying*
Ear tugging and crying are typical signs of otitis media.

E. *Symmetrical burns on the hands*
Symmetrical burns are indicative of physical abuse.

43. The nurse is caring for a client who had a thoracotomy 48 hours ago and now has left lower lobe chest tubes. The nurse notes that a chest tube is not tidaling. Which action should the nurse take first?

Rationales:

A. *Check for kinks in the chest drainage system*
Normal fluctuation of the water, called tidaling, reflects the intrapleural pressure during inspiration and expiration. If no tidaling is observed (rising with inspiration and falling with expiration in a spontaneously breathing patient), the drainage system may be blocked. An absence of fluctuation may mean that the lung has fully re-expanded or can mean that there is an obstruction in the chest tube. A simple step is to ensure that there are no kinks that would occlude the chest tube and prevent lung drainage and expansion

B. *Assess the heart rate and blood pressure*
Checking the heart rate and blood pressure is not directly related to the lack of chest tube drainage

C. *Notify the rapid response team immediately*
Although the nurse should immediately notify the Rapid Response Team for tracheal deviation, sudden onset of dyspnea or mediastinal shift, the absence of tidaling may not be a medical emergency.

D. *Momentarily disconnect from wall suction*
Disconnecting the chest tube from wall suction will not affect tidaling or the water seal.

44. While the nurse is caring for a client who has had an MI, the monitor alarm sounds and the nurse notes ventricular fibrillation. What should be the nurse's first course of action?

Rationales:

A. *Notify the healthcare provider*
This may be an appropriate action after assessment of the client's clinical status.

B. *Increase the oxygen concentration*
This may be an appropriate action after assessment of the client's clinical status.

C. *Assess the client's level of consciousness*
If a monitor alarm sounds, the nurse should first assess the client's clinical status to see whether the problem is an actual dysrhythmia or a monitoring system malfunction.

D. *Prepare to defibrillate the client*
This may be an appropriate action after assessment of the client's clinical status.

45. The physician has prescribed the removal of a client's internal jugular central line catheter. To remove the catheter safely, the nurse should give which intervention(s) the highest priority? (Select all that apply.)

Rationales:

A. *Carefully remove the Bioderm dressing*
Removing the Bioderm dressing is important, but it is not a safety priority.

B. *Place the client in the Trendelenburg position*
The procedure for removing the catheter safely is (1) place the client in the Trendelenburg position; (2) have the client take a deep breath and hold it; and (3) gently withdraw the catheter while applying direct pressure with sterile gauze. Holding the breath creates positive pressure in the intrathoracic space, and the Trendelenburg position minimizes the risk of air entering the catheter.

C. *Send the catheter tip to the lab for a C & S*
The catheter tip may or may not be sent to the lab, depending on the protocol of the facility.

D. *Have the client take a deep breath during removal*
The procedure for removing the catheter safely is (1) place the client in the Trendelenburg position; (2) have the client take a deep breath and hold it; and (3) gently withdraw the catheter while applying direct pressure with sterile gauze. Holding the breath creates positive pressure in the intrathoracic space, and the Trendelenburg position minimizes the risk of air entering the catheter.

E. *Apply pressure for 20 minutes after removal of the catheter*
Applying pressure for 20 minutes is a technique used in arterial line withdrawal to prevent bleeding.